Anaesthesia:
A Concise Handbook

Anaesthesia:
A Concise Handbook

Graham Arthurs
Consultant Anaesthetist
Maelor Hospital
Wrexham

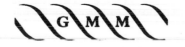

LONDON • SAN FRANCISCO

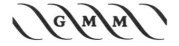

© 2001

Greenwich Medical Media Limited
137 Euston Road
London
NW1 2AA

870 Market Street, Ste 720,
San Francisco,
CA 94102

ISBN 1 84110 080 3

First Published 2001

A catalogue record for this book is available from the British Library.

Typeset by Charon Tec Pvt. Ltd, Chennai, India

Printed in the UK by the Alden Group

Distributed by Plymbridge Distributors Ltd and
in the USA by Jamco Distribution

Visit our website at www.greenwich-medical.co.uk

Contents

Preface

Anaesthesia requires the practitioner to respond rapidly to many situations. The trainee anaesthetist is required to accumulate a wealth of knowledge in order to know what they can safely offer and when they should refer for more help. The experienced practitioner needs to keep up to date. Safety and standards demand that we practice within guidelines and protocols, which have been recommended by different professional bodies.

This concise handbook includes guidelines, protocols and the outline for many practical situations and procedures. There are many items that might be considered general knowledge or common sense but are often not remembered or explained.

In this pocket sized book many pieces of information have been brought together that have been collected over years of clinical practice. Some ideas are handed down by word of mouth, some have appeared as letters or are in reviews and textbooks but their importance may be lost amongst the wealth of other information.

We are all faced with information over load. This handbook aims to bring together helpful information for safe and effective every day practice. The anaesthetic trainee has many different specialist texts to consult and this handbook is no substitute for such bench books. It is hoped it will give guidance for the management of life threatening emergencies and hints for dealing with difficult situations.

The trainer who is looking for topics for in service training in theatre will find many ideas that can be used as a basis for further explanation and discussion. Just as this information is required for safe practice so the same areas are often the subjects of questions in postgraduate examinations. It is also hoped that as knowledge is updated the pages will become annotated with personal notes of individual's guidelines and hints, which is where this book started, as personal notes of the author.

The handbook is a quick reference for topics including:

- outline procedures for common clinical situations, including airway management and local blocks

- protocols and guidelines for cardiac resuscitation and many other emergencies, as available in 2001

- quick reference interpretation of ECG and CXR

- explanations for practice based on physiological principles

- tables of drugs and physiological parameters

Graham Arthurs
July 2001

Acknowledgements

Tony Bailey for Illustrations.

Mary McKeon and Richard Bailey for library assistance.

My family for support during the preparation of the text.

Gavin Smith for advice in preparing the manuscript.

Airway

Normal airway

The normal airway remains patent due to the tension in the muscles supporting the larynx. The strap muscles, sternohyoid and sternothyroid link the larynx to the sternum while stylohyoid, hyoglossus, mylohyoid, geniohyoid and digastric link the larynx to the skull and the mandible which in turn is held by masseter to the skull. Any loss of tension in these muscles due to sleep, alcohol, illness, sedative or analgesic drugs may lead to an obstruction at some part of the airway: tongue on palate, tongue on posterior pharyngeal wall, epiglottis on posterior pharyngeal wall or onto laryngeal inlet.

To create a clear airway:

- Place the fingers behind the angle of the mandible and force the chin forward – jaw thrust. Most people breathe through their nose so the mouth does not need to be open.

- Neck flexed and head extended – sniffing the morning air. Use two pillows to support the head.

- Guedel airway: *Adult.* Airway length – distance from the angle of the mouth to the angle of the mandible gives the airway length, not including the bite-block length, or from mid-point of lips (incisors) to mandible angle if bite block is included. Hold so that the apex of the curve that will pass over the tongue is facing the lower lip. The first movement passes the tip of the airway between the teeth and up into the space of the hard palate. Then gently corkscrew the airway, rotating through 180° and push forward over the tongue. The proximal end is the flattened bite block with a reinforced core to prevent obstruction by biting. An airway which is too long will irritate the pharynx, leading to coughing and breath holding.

Children. The airway can be passed directly into the mouth without rotation. This avoids trauma to the palatal mucosa.

- A short bite block or a child's airway in an adult is useful to prevent biting a tracheal tube and prevent apposition of the teeth without provoking a gag reflex.[1]

- A thick suture can be attached to the flange and taped to the cheek for safety when the airway is small for the size of the mouth.[2]

Masks

- To obtain a seal between the face with a beard, or any other deformity, and a face mask, a pad of conductive gel as used under a defibrillator pad is useful. Cut a hole in the centre to fit the airway.[3]

- A tracheostomy can be difficult to cover with a mask. An upside down Randell Baker mask fits tightly over the stoma[4] (see Figure 6, page 15).

- A size 5 mask can be used turned through 180° and fitted over the mouth. Three acromegalic patients could not be ventilated with a size 5 mask. The mask is turned round and the cushion either obstructs the nose or an ODA pinches the nose shut for ventilation.[5]

Variable performance masks

- Variable performance masks mix the oxygen flow with air during inspiration. If the mask fits too closely to the face it limits inspiration. Patient comfort and compliance improves if some part is cut to make bigger side openings or a hole made in the top of the mask. This increases arterial oxygen saturations by 3–8% and possibly allows better carbon dioxide elimination.[6]

- The increase in oxygen can be calculated by making a number of assumptions.

If inspiration lasts for 1 s, oxygen flowing at 6 l/min will deliver 100 ml in 1 s. If the tidal volume is 600 ml, then 100 ml of oxygen will be added. This leaves $600 - 100 = 500$ ml of air, of which 20% (100 ml) is oxygen. So inspiratory oxygen is now 200 in 600 ml or 33%.

- Some masks are called ventimasks but do not work on a venturi principle. They have variable performance.

Fixed performance masks

- Fixed performance masks are fitted with a venturi device so that the oxygen entrains a fixed ratio of air before it enters the mask.

- These masks will deliver the fixed oxygen concentration stated on the mask providing the flow of the mixture of oxygen and air exceeds the peak inspiratory flow rate (PIFR) of about 35 l/min. The mask gives a minimum oxygen flow rate to achieve this PIFR.

- These are used when a fixed oxygen concentration is important. Patients with type II respiratory failure (blue bloaters) have a respiratory drive that is part low oxygen and part high carbon dioxide tension. The hypoxic drive to respiration will be reduced if the inspired oxygen tension is raised too much.

One hundred per cent oxygen mask has a reservoir into which oxygen is fed. The patient breathes in 100% oxygen and breathes out to air.

Laryngeal mask airway

- Insertion requires suppression of the laryngeal reflexes, particularly those associated with the tenth cranial nerve.

- The cuff should be deflated and curved back on itself.

- The tip should be well lubricated on the palatal surface.

- It is passed so that the tip slides along the palate and into the oropharynx until it lodges against the superior pharyngeal constrictor.

- It is doubtful that cricoid pressure can be effectively maintained with this airway.

- While not making a seal with the larynx IPPV is possible and the larygeal muscles will contract in expiration to create a positive pressure.

Laryngeal mask sizes

Size	Patient	Volume (ml)
1	Neonate	4
1½		7
2	Child	10
2½		14
3	30–50 kg	20
4	Adult	30
5		40

Pre-use check

- Lumen clear, tube transparent, secure connector.

- Flexion to 180° causes no kink.

- Cuff should hold volume +50% without herniation.

- Use no more than 40 times.

Insertion

- Suppress laryngeal reflexes.

- Neck flexed, head extended.

- Gloved hand with index finger along the concave surface at junction of cuff and tube.

- Lubricate only back (palatal) surface.

- Press tip flat against the hard palate and continue backward pressure to pass behind the epiglottis.

- Only pass index finger into mouth.
- Check whether black line faces upper lip.
- Inflate cuff to 60 cmH$_2$O.
- Connect gas supply, insert bite block, fix tube.

Airway management device

Airway management device is an oral tube airway with two cuffs. A smaller distal cuff seals at the upper oesophageal. A larger proximal cuff fills the oropharynx.

Sizes: 3–3.5 for 30–60 kg; 4–5 for >60 kg.

Teeth

Check for loose teeth in

- children loosing deciduous teeth,
- patients with poor dental hygiene and gum disease,
- odd teeth with gaps.

Options

- A full gum shield may restrict access during intubation.
- A gum shield with outer wings removed. The central part will protect the teeth while leaving better access for a tracheal tube.[7]
- Create a personalised, thin gum shield with aluminium foil.
- For loose teeth or an isolated peg tooth, dental departments have a range of materials that can be used to make a tailor made tooth guard, in about 10 min.
- The flange on the blade of a Macintosh laryngoscope can be fitted with a strip of thin (2 mm thick) polyfoam, 1 cm wide and 3–4 cm long, to provide a cushion for teeth and gums.[8,9]

If there is a loose tooth consider threading a silk tie through the interdental clefts and tie a knot at the base of the tooth. The thread is taped to the side of the face until the end of the procedure. If the tooth is dislodged it can be retrieved at the end of the thread.[10]

A common complaint against anaesthetists is dental damage. If a tooth is displaced and lost at intubation and there is airway obstruction consider the Heimlick manoeuvre. Stand behind patient and compress the abdomen below the xiphisternum, or the lower chest. For small children, hold head down and slap on back. Then take

- chest X-ray,
- fibre-optic laryngoscopy – bronchoscope,
- rigid bronchoscopy if above the carina,
- oesophagoscopy.

Tell patient it may be passed in the stools if in GI tract.

Dentures

- Anaesthetists' views differ as to whether dentures should be removed preoperatively.
- Advantages of leaving well-fitting dentures in place until after induction of anaesthesia: application of the mask and maintenance of an airway easier; patient is less distressed and more able to communicate; the alveolar gum margin is less likely to be damaged by the laryngoscope; many patients sleep with their dentures; may protect isolated teeth from further damage.
- Disadvantages: these concern that the denture will become detached during laryngoscopy; inhalation of a full denture must be very difficult.
- Compromise: remove it in the anaesthetic room just before or after laryngoscopy.[11–13]

Laryngoscopy

Laryngoscope blade

- A straight blade (Magill) with no thickening at the tip, passes behind the epiglottis and lifts it up. Uses: floppy epiglottis particularly in children, inadequate hyo-epiglottic ligament. The under surface of the epiglottis is innervated by the vagus nerve which might be stimulated during the manoeuvre.

- The Macintosh blade, with a rounded end, passes into the vallecula. The handle is lifted up to the ceiling. It is not used to rotate the blade on the incisor teeth, which will turn the larynx anteriorly and away from view.

- A polio blade fits to the handle with an obtuse angle. Originally used for patients with chest plaster casts but has a place whenever the neck cannot be extended or the chest and sternum are prominent.

- A laryngoscope has been designed with a blade that has two curves of 20° and 30° and widens at the distal end to lift the epiglottis. There is no vertical flange to damage the incisor teeth. The wide flat shaft presses the tongue down.[14]

- The brightness of the light is limited by the 3 V battery power. Batteries should be replaced every month and should be removed if the handle is not used. Corroded batteries are difficult to remove from the handle. The bulb will burn brighter at the end of its life as the filament becomes thin. The fibre-optic bundles in blades break when dropped and autoclaved. The blades fitted with fibre-optic bundles give a reduced light over a period of use.

- An optically powered laryngoscope handle (Rimmer Brothers) gives consistently more light over a greater area than battery operated handles.[15]

Local anaesthetic technique for procedures on the larynx, including intubation:

- Anticholinegic IV to reduce secretions and prevent bradycardia. In the sitting position ask the patient to protrude the tongue and grasp it with a swab. The patient takes a deep inspiration and maximum expiration. Then spray 5 puffs of lidocaine spray (lignocaine 5×10 mg) into the pharynx. Patient breathes in, gargles and is asked to wash the remaining fluid over the tongue. Repeat a second time. Spray 2–3 puffs into each nostril. Choose the left nostril first to avoid trauma of the turbinates. Maximum adult dose of lidocaine is 3 mg/kg or 20 puffs of 10 mg.

Intubation

- The head should be extended at the atlanto-occipital joint and the neck flexed. This is achieved by supporting the head on pillows or an inflated 1 l bag.

- The Macintosh curved blade is designed to fit the vallecula and by forward lift raise the hyoid cartilage, stretch the hyo-epiglottic ligament and hence lift the epiglottis. If the epiglottis is not lifted by this indirect approach the blade tip, or a straight Magill blade, needs to go under the epiglottis and lifts it directly. The other hand is used to clear the lips from between the scope and the teeth and then to manipulate the thyroid cartilage to line up the larynx with the scope.

Cricoid pressure

- Sellick (a London anaesthetist) described pressure on the cricoid cartilage pressing back on the C5 cervical vertebra if the neck is extended, to reduce regurgitation. With a pillow behind the head and the neck flexed pressure will often be against C6.

The amount of pressure required is described as 44 Newtons (N), which causes pain when applied to the nasal bridge. In reality pressures of 10–120 N are applied; 40 N offers 50% of patients protection against regurgitation and 66 N protects 83%.[16] These pressures are painful if applied to the awake patient, so effective pressure can only be applied once awareness has been lost.

- Cricoid pressure can distort the laryngeal anatomy and make intubation difficult by rotating the larynx anteriorly. This effect can be reduced by placing a hand behind the neck to provide support during cricoid pressure or by using a pillow 27 cm long × 10 cm wide × 5 cm high behind the neck.[17]

Tracheal tubes

- The cuff pressure should be sufficient to prevent the passage of fluid but not cause mucosal ischaemia. Low pressure, high volume cuffs cause a dynamic seal during inflation by back-pressure of gas in the trachea, but no seal during expiration.

- The use of a syringe to inflate the cuff often produces over inflation.[18] When cuff pressure exceeds mucosal perfusion pressure at 20–35 mmHg ischaemia occurs. Cuff pressure will increase during the administration of nitrous oxide.

To prevent a rise in cuff pressure:

- A three-way tap connected to the pilot tube is connected through manometer tubing to a pressure gauge (Portex). The cuff pressure can be read and adjusted from time to time.[19]

- To prevent the increase in cuff pressure due to nitrous oxide, fill the cuff with gas from the breathing circuit or with water.[20]

- A manometer column of fluid is set at about 25 cmH$_2$O. Tubing is attached to the pilot tube by a three-way tap and the cuff inflated until the fluid reaches the desired height.[21,22]

Tracheal tube length in adults

> Adult incisor to carina distance: 24–29 cm.
> Oral tube length: male – 23 cm
>   female – 21 cm.
> Teeth to mid-trachea =
> (height (cm)/10) + 2.
> Nasal tube length: external nares to mid-trachea = (height (cm)/10) + 8.
> Child oral tube length =
> (age (years)/2) + 12.
> Nasal tube length = (age (years)/2) + 15.
> Preformed tubes: The correct length may take precedence over the diameter.

- The distance from incisors to carina varies from 24 to 29 cm in adults. The distance from the radial border of the second to the ulnar border of fifth metacarpo-phalangeal joint (knuckle distance) × 2.5 is equal to the distance from the incisors to just above the carina where the tip of the tube can rest.[23]

- Securing the oral tracheal tube at the incisor teeth or gums at the 23 cm mark in men and 21 cm mark in women of average adult build reduces the likelihood of endobronchial intubation.[24]

- The distance from the vocal cords to the carina in adults is 12.1–12.6 cm. Ideally the tip of the trachea tube should be at the mid-point of the trachea. The average distance from the site of the proximal bonding of the cuff to the tube, to the tip of the tube, in tubes 7–9 mm ID, is 7.5 cm (6.5–8.5). This means that the tip of the tube will usually lie within 5 cm of the carina.[25]

- The relationship between the patient's height and the dimensions of the upper airway can be defined to create formulae for predicting the appropriate length of tracheal tubes.

- Oral tube: teeth to mid-trachea = (height (cm)/10) + 2.

- Nasal tube: external naris to mid-point of trachea = (height (cm)/10) + 8.[26]

The trachea is likely to shorten during anaesthesia due to

- reduction in FRC by 20% due to loss of nitrogen from lung,

- pressure from abdominal contents, Trendelenburg position, lithotomy, laproscopic gas or packs.

The distal tube can then pass into the right bronchus, even if it was in the trachea at the start of the anaesthetic.

Tracheal tube length in children

- Oral tube: (age (years)/2) + 12 cm.

- Nasal tube: (age (years)/2) + 15 cm.

- The analysis of tube length used in 634 children who were underweight but had no airway pathology showed a good agreement with the formulae:

- Internal diameter: (16 + age (years))/4 mm.

- Length: (3 × internal diameter (mm)) + 2 cm.

- The reduced weight of these children did not influence the length calculated by this formula.[27]

- Tube length can be estimated as twice the distance from the angle of the mouth to the tragus in children and one and a half this distance in adults.

- Most anaesthetists cut the tube to a predetermined length according to

a formula.[28] An alternative is to insert an uncut tube nasally. When in position the tube is cut halfway across its lumen, the connector is inserted while holding the proximal end. Once the connector is in place the remaining piece is removed.[29]

Diameter

The internal diameter of a tube is the one quoted. The thickness of most tubes increases with size and varies between manufacturers. So the 4.0 mm ID will be 5.4 mm OD Portex (polar) up to 6.1 mm for the Rusch reinforced. The 5 mm ID will not be just 1 mm bigger, but an OD of 6.8 mm Portex (polar) up to 7.5 mm Rusch (reinforced). In practice one tube may fit comfortably; increasing to the next size may be a traumatic fit.[30] The length of preformed tubes increases with increase in diameter. As length seems to be constant for age the diameter should be determined by the length for a preformed tube.

Cuff leaks

Accidental deflation of a tracheal tube cuff can be managed as follows:

- Pack the pharynx with gauze wet with tap water (saline or dextrose will dehydrate the mucosa).

- The pilot tube of a bronchial cuff can be connected to an empty 3 l infusion bag which is inflated to keep the pressure at about 8 kPa for small perforations.[31]

- A slowly leaking cuff can be inflated with oxygen from a cylinder. A manometer is necessary to prevent over inflation. This will only work for small perforations. In a microperforated Portex cuff, 0.5 kPa could be maintained with a flow rate of 1 l/min, 1.5 kPa with a flow rate of 5 l/min.[32]

Confirmation of tracheal intubation

- Auscultation with a stethoscope over both axillae and stomach is the oldest and cheapest means of detecting correct placement of a tube in the trachea and not in the oesophagus.[33]

- The absence of condensation in a PVC tube reliably indicates oesophageal intubation. The presence of condensation is not a specific indicator of tube position as up to 100% of oesophageal intubations can have condensation in the tube.[34]

- Palpate the tube and arytenoids with a gloved finger.

- Capnography identifies carbon dioxide from the lungs. A carbon dioxide detector may give a false positive for tracheal intubation if it detects carbon dioxide in the stomach after the patient has drunk a fizzy drink, taken alkalis for indigestion,[35,36] or expired gas has been blown into the stomach while ventilating using a mask.

The oesophageal detector

- The ability to recover air injected into the trachea but not from the oesophagus was first described in 1980.[37]

- The use of air from a 60 ml syringe injected into a tracheal tube was later taken up by Wee. If the tube is in the trachea the air can be drawn back, if it is in the oesophagus the air cannot be drawn back.[38,39] The test has been claimed to be reliable with no false positives in 100 cases.[40] The passage of 50 ml of air may not be reliable in patients with upper or lower airway obstruction or with low lung compliance[41] and in children the reliability of air injection has been questioned.[42] If the cuff is overinflated air may not be drawn back.

- In an emergency place a filter on the tracheal tube and blow air down the tracheal tube, both to resuscitate the

patient and to listen for air returning to confirm correct placement of the tube.

One problem with making a detector from an evacuator is the development of a significant negative pressure which could lead to airway collapse in patients with increased airway pressure e.g. asthma. This may lead to a false negative result. A 60 ml syringe has the advantage of exerting a gentle aspiration.[43]

Position of the tube cuff

Palpating the trachea between the cricoid cartilage and sternal notch by holding it between index finger and thumb can be used to determine two things about a tracheal tube:

- If the cuff is inflated and deflated while palpating the trachea the cuff will be felt to expand and contract. If this is not felt the trachea tube is either below the sternal notch and in too far or in the larynx or mouth. Feeling the cuff does not differentiate between tracheal and oesophageal intubation.[44,45]

- Rolling the trachea or cricoid cartilage under the fingers from side to side will be felt like two tubes if the oesophagus has been intubated. If the tube is in the trachea only one tube will be felt as the cricoid cartilage cannot be rolled on a tube in the trachea.[46]

A nasogastric tube passed through the tracheal tube can be used in three ways to detect oesophageal intubation.

- If it is in the oesophagus over 40 cm will pass.

- When suction is applied the mucosal wall limits the suction and the tube cannot be easily withdrawn.

- Bile coloured fluid may be aspirated.[47]

A 16G suction catheter or (Yankauer catheter) can be used to intubate the trachea when the larynx is narrowed.[48]

Tracheal tube fixation

Tape and knot

- To secure a tracheal tube, a knot that does not slip is required. The constrictor knot, which will hold a boa constrictor, is one such knot[49] (Figure 1).

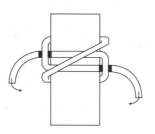

Final knot

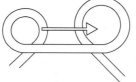

Step 1

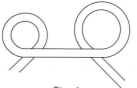

Step 2

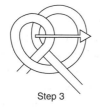

Step 3

Figure 1 – Constrictor knot.

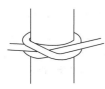

Figure 2 – Clove hitch.

- The clove hitch is a simple knot that can be loosely placed and then tightened after correct placement of the tube. The knot can be loosened and retightened a number of times[50] (Figure 2).

Tape

- Sticking tape should be used with caution as it may cause an allergic reaction or remove a variable amount of the epidermis when pulled away. The child's and delicate facial skin can be protected by painting with tinct. benz. co. Elastoplast will hold to the tube and to the skin. If there is allergy a hypoallergenic plaster is used.

- Adhesive tape may not adhere well to silicone tubes. Once the tube is in place a length of strong surgical silk is wound around the tube and tied tightly to provide a firm attachment for tape.[51]

The tracheal tube can be made more receptive to ties by the application of

- *self-locking STA-STRAP cable* ties fixed and tightened around the tracheal tube where the connector is inserted,[52]

- *O rings* will fix to the tracheal tube connector.[53]

Fixing small tubes

- Paint the skin with tinct. benz. co. and apply 1 cm wide tape.

- The tracheal tube may kink at the teeth, particularly when hidden under drapes. A 2.5 mm Portex tube, which has an outside diameter of 3.4 mm, can be reinforced in the mouth by fitting a 3.5 mm tube over it, cut so that 4 cm of the 2.5 mm tube is uncovered at the distal end.[54]

- At the mouth, an infant size 1 anaesthetic mask is modified by cutting a square hole 15 × 15 cm to fit the tracheal tube. After intubation the mask is slipped over the tube and the mask is fixed to the face with adhesive tape.[55]

- A method to secure a tracheal tube in infants with mid-line facial defects: The child is intubated. A hole is made at the centre of a 5 in. × 5 in. piece of triple thickness kitchen plastic wrap. The hole in the wrap is slid over the tube and the wrap pushed into the crevices of the oral and nasal cavities leaving a rim outside the mouth. Liquid silicone foam is directed onto the wrap so that a mould is formed in the mouth, encasing the tube.[56]

Intubation

Normal airway
Head on two pillows sniffing the
  morning air
Preoxygenate with 6–10 deep breaths
Detect tube in trachea by
 – Stethoscope listen over axillae and
   stomach
 – Capnograph

Difficult airway above mandible, facial injury
Preoxygenate, cricoid pressure
No IV sedation/muscle relaxant before
  manual ventilation
Inhalation induction – intubate or
  fibre optic intubation, cricothyroid
  puncture, minitracheostomy
Tuohy needle and retrograde epidural
  catheter through cricothyroid
  membrane

Difficult airway below mandible,
neck injury or swelling
Preoxygenate, cricoid pressure not
  reliable
No IV sedation/muscle relaxant before
  manual ventilation
Small diameter tube or catheter available
Awake LA fibre-optic intubation
Inhalation induction, oral or blind nasal
  intubation
McCoy laryngoscope

Failed intubation
Oxygen by mask, manual ventilation until
  spontaneous ventilation
Release cricoid pressure – may give a
  better view of the larynx
Try bougie, laryngeal mask, airway
  management device, fibre-optic
  intubation
Wake up or if urgent anaesthesia: LA and
  IV drugs midazolam, ketamine,
  anticholinergic, prokinetic agent
  metoclopramide or cricothyroid
  puncture to oxygenate

Aids to intubating a narrow larynx

Alternatives to tracheal tube: Foley catheter, tracheal suction catheter, Yankauer suction tube.

- When the opening to the trachea is narrow a small diameter (<5 mm ID) tracheal tube is needed. These are paediatric tubes and may be too short for an adult.

- A Foley catheter can be used for intubating the small, narrow opening to a larynx, where only a slit is seen, often with a bubble of froth at the opening. Introduce by holding with Magill forceps. Pass so that the catheter balloon lies just below the cords. A length of intravenous extension tubing is attached to the balloon port. Fifteen litres of fresh gas flow are attached to the catheter to ventilate the lungs. If there is a leak of gas through the larynx the balloon is distended during inspiration. When the balloon is deflated expiration occurs. The catheter balloon is robust enough to maintain inflation and deflation for a period of time.[57] If there is no leak the gas flow should be intermittent.

- A tracheal suction catheter or a Yankauer suction tube with greater rigidity can be used to secure a difficult airway.[58]

- All these catheters can have oxygen fitted to the lumen while they are passed.

Difficult airway (Table 1)

Never give a drug that may cause apnoea if the airway cannot be maintained.

Predict a difficult airway. Examine patient sitting.

- Obese, short, immobile neck. Prominent incisors, receding mandible with no obvious angle or obtuse angle.

- Mouth should open to admit three fingers between upper and lower incisors.

- A history of snoring, obstructive sleep apnoea, previous difficulty. A difficult airway often means a difficult intubation.

- Thyromental distance normally over 6 cm or three fingers.

- Finger on chin should rise above finger on occiput when neck extends.

Check lateral X-ray of the neck in extension and flexion.

- Visible with mouth open: Class 1 tonsillar fauces and pillars. Class 2 uvula and soft palate. Class 3 soft palate and base of uvula. Class 4 only tongue and hard palate. Classes 3 and 4 are possibly difficult to intubate (Mallampti et al.).[59]

Apparatus for a difficult airway

Nasal

Use a vasoconstrictor e.g. ephedrine, lubrication, use left nostril to reduce trauma as the pointed end of the tube is on the right it will slide past the turbinates on the left.

- A nasopharyngeal airway passed alone or as an introducer for a Foley catheter with a flow of 2–3 l/min oxygen attached.

Table 1 – Difficult airway

Unexpected		Expected (consider two anaesthetists)	
Unable to oxygenate	Able to oxygenate	Local anaesthetic	Inhalation induction
Call for help	Call for help	Awake	Asleep
Narrow larynx try suction catheter through larynx	Face mask	Problem	
	Oral or nasal airway	Above mandible	Below mandible
	Laryngeal mask	Cricothyroid puncture	Secure airway first,
Vallecular cyst push out of way or puncture	Combi tube	or Tuohy needle and	cricoid pressure unreliable
	Consider intubation with bougie alone	catheter possible	
Cricothyroid puncture 14/16G cannula with oxygen via green tubing from cylinder or common gas outlet	Bougie through a laryngeal mask airway		
	Wake up if not urgent	Preoxygenate	
	Epidural catheter via Tuohy needle in cricothyroid membrane	Prokinetic agent – Metoclopramide	
		Drying agent – Glycopyrronium	
		N/G tube pass and remove	
	Fibre-optic intubation	LA to nose and oropharynx	
		Fibre-optic intubation: oral or nasal tube	
		Blind nasal intubation	

Urgent operation
LA infiltration or regional technique
Ketamine 0.5 mg/kg IV repeat with
- Midazolam 1–10 mg
- Glycopyrronium 300 μg
- Oxygen mask 4–6 l/min
N/G tube to empty stomach
Prokinetic agent – Metoclopramide 10 mg IV

- A cuffed nasopharyngeal tube passed through the nostril[60,61] and the cuff inflated in the pharynx.

Oral

- Laryngeal mask airway

- *Combi tube*: Double lumen tube passed blindly. It either enters the trachea and the distal cuff is inflated; or more likely it enters the oesophagus and both cuffs are inflated in the oesophagus and pharynx. Air then passes from the outer tube through holes in the wall into the pharynx and hence into the larynx.

Facial hair

- A sheet of transparent dressing with a hole at the centre can be applied over the tube to fix to tube and around the mouth and nasal area.[62]

- When there is more than 1 cm of moustache hair the tube and hair can be taped tightly together. There is 1 cm of movement in the tube but it is securely fixed to the face.[63]

When the patient is allergic to tape, has much facial hair or tape will not hold due to injury, a length of oxygen tubing is cut into 42–47 cm for adults, 35–40 cm for small adults and 25–30 cm for children. A double strand of umbilical tape is pulled through the oxygen tube lumen and knotted at each end of the tube. The oxygen tubing is placed around the nape of the neck and the tracheal tube secured by the tapes.[64] This will prevent the tape cutting into the neck.

Difficult intubation

- The Mallampati score,[59] alerts anaesthetists to some 50% of difficult intubations.

- If the lower incisors cannot be brought edge to edge with the upper incisors

(Class C mandibular protrusion) then a difficult intubation is invariable, especially with cervical disease.[65]

- A sternomental distance of 12.5 cm or less is a reliable indicator of difficult intubation.[66]

- Thyromental distance (TMD) is an indicator of difficult intubation. The TMD varied from 3.5 to 9 cm in 250 patients. Less than 6 cm predicted 60% of difficult laryngoscopies but just 25% of easy ones. Only 10% of predicted difficult laryngoscopies proved to be difficult; 6.5 cm or more cannot be taken to signify an easy laryngoscopy.[67]

- When TMD is used to predict difficult intubation the reason for the shortening should also be considered. The TMD will be shortened if the head will not extend, if the mandible is receding or if the larynx is high.[68]

- When the space between chest and chin is short consider using a polio blade or turning and lowering the laryngoscope handle towards the side of the neck. Then insert the blade laterally from the right or left side of the mouth and rotate the handle as the blade is passed over the tongue[69] (Figure 3), or remove the blade from the handle of the laryngoscope. Pass the blade and then re-attach the handle once the blade is in the mouth.[70]

- A tubular laryngoscope introduced from the right side of the mouth has an

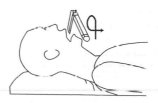

Figure 3 – Blade introduced from right side of mouth.

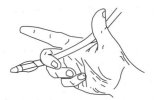

Figure 4 – Tube held like chopstick.

advantage when the incisors are prominent and when there are gaps between the teeth. It can then be used to pass an introducer before a tracheal tube. Pilling instruments make a split scope for paediatric use. The laryngoscope splits down the centre. The two halves are held together by a quick release screw.[71]

- Intubation may be made quicker by holding the tracheal tube like a chopstick in the middle, ring and little fingers, so that the thumb and index finger are free to open the mouth (Figure 4). After partial insertion of the laryngoscope the tracheal tube is introduced along the inner wall of the right cheek. The laryngoscope is advanced and the epiglottis lifted almost at the same time as the tracheal tube is advanced through the cords.[72]

- A gum elastic bougie reduces dental damage and can be passed towards the larynx when it is out of view but its position can be estimated. The tube is rail-roaded over the bougie but the tip is likely to lodge on the right vocal cords. It is advisable to rotate the tube through at least 90° anticlockwise to avoid the arytenoids[73–75] or use a continuous rotating motion to introduce the tube through the larynx. Once in place the bougie will only pass 30 cm or so if it is in a bronchus. If in the oesophagus it will pass its whole length of 60 cm.[76]

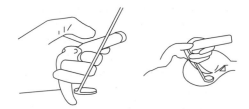

Figure 5 – Use of ENT mirror to see larynx indirectly.

- For an indirect view of the hidden larynx a long bladed ENT mirror is placed in the oropharynx with the handle on the right of the mouth (Figure 5). The mirror is best held in place by an assistant while a bougie is passed into the larynx.[77]

Introducers

- The gum elastic bougie is essential in any difficult intubation. If the bougie is in the trachea it will pass some 30 cm, if in the oesophagus it will pass its whole length of 60 cm. Once the bougie is in the trachea the tracheal tube is rail-roaded over, rotating anticlockwise to pass through the cords.

- A smaller diameter introducer can be made from a Fogarty embolectomy catheter that has a soft tip, is long and is marked in cm. A 4.5 mm tracheal tube will pass easily over the catheter.[78]

- To remove a mucus plug a Foley catheter, or other slim catheter with balloon, will pass by a mucus plug, the balloon inflated with water and then used to pull the mucus out.[79]

- A tracheal tube can be given additional angle to the curve by placing a stylet into the tube from the tracheal end and bending the stylet into a J. After 20 min the stylet is removed to leave the tube in its new shape.[80]

- A difficult intubation in a 2.8 kg neonate, too small for a fibre-optic laryngoscope, used a 3 mm ID Portex tube passed down the right nostril to act as a nasopharyngeal airway to provide oxygen and volatile agent. A ureteric catheter Ch 4 was passed through the tracheal tube and into the larynx to act as a guide for passing the tracheal tube. An alternative is to pass the guide through the suction port of the fibrescope but this means removing the fibrescope before achieving intubation.[81]

- A flexible guide wire passes into the tracheal, under direct vision, through the suction channel of the endoscope. The scope is removed and an appropriate size of uretheral or renal dilator passed over the wire. A 6 mm tube passes over the dilator into the trachea.[82]

Nasal intubation

Techniques to guide the tube atraumatically through the nose and to avoid material becoming caught in the lumen.

- Use the left nostril so that the point of the tube passes along the septum, not against the tubinates.

- To prevent trauma and blockage of the tube a 16 FG Jaques or Foley catheter[83,84] can be used as an introducer, pushed beyond the distal end of the tube. The balloon is inflated (with saline to reduce bulging caused by air) until it forms a smooth taper with the end of the tube.[85]

- The tip of the tube may become stuck on the arytenoid or above the vocal cord. If the tube is rotated through 90° anticlockwise rather than clockwise it passes without further difficulty. The introducer should be rotated as well.[86]

Doughty blade and REA tubes in ENT operations

The REA preformed south facing tubes, without the advantage of a reinforced proximal connection, may become trapped in the grove in the Doughty blade of the Boyle Davies gag. This may kink and obstruct the tube or trap the tube which can only be removed when the gag is removed. To remove the gag means extubating the patient. The gag can be modified by the addition of tape or a stainless steel bar $18 \times 4 \times 1$ mm to the convex surface of the blade at the mid-point of the slot.[87]

Blind nasal intubation

- *Local anaesthetic spray*. Breathing spontaneously makes it easier to hear the tube nearing the larynx. The head is placed sniffing the morning air, on two pillows. The left hand passes a well-lubricated, small volume cuff, tracheal tube, into the left nostril while the right hand holds the occiput with thumb pushing the mandible forward.

- In the left nostril the nasal tube has the bevel directed laterally so as to pass the leading edge away from the turbinates. In this way the turbinates are not damaged. The proximal end of the tube is pulled cephalad to direct the bevel along the floor of the nasal cavity and below the inferior turbinate. Once the tip has passed the uvula the part of the tube out of the nose is given its normal curvature and advanced into the larynx.[88]

- If it sticks watch where the tube pushes against the anterior neck and rotate the tube to keep to the mid-line. Flex the head with the right hand or guide the tube into the larynx by placing the index and middle fingers over the tongue.

- One key to success for awake nasal intubation is to follow the maximum breath sound. This is made easier if a stethoscope is attached to the proximal end of the tube while it is passed through the oropharynx to amplify the noise of breathing. A side stream analyser T piece is one way of making the connection.[89,90] As well as the stethoscope a capnograph can be attached to the nasotracheal tube.

- The cuff of the nasal tube can be partly inflated in the nasopharynx and the tube advanced until resistance is encountered. Prewarming the tube may reduce trauma during the introduction.[91]

Nasal intubation – children

- Nasopharyngeal secretions are common in children. The tracheal tube can be obstructed by these secretions which it picks up in transit through the nasal passage. Direct suction to the nasal canal leads to oedema, trauma and possible bleeding. A better approach is to pass a thinner catheter through the tracheal tube and use it to keep the tube patent, as a bougie and if needed as an introducer.[92] Suction can be applied to the nasopharynx from behind the soft palate under direct laryngoscopy once intubation has been performed.[93]

Fibre-optically assisted intubation

- *Sitting or lying*. Sitting allows secretions to flow out of the pharynx and may be more comfortable for the kyphoscoliotic patient. Anticholinergic to dry secretions. Draw the tongue forward with a swab. Ask the patient to breath in and then deeply out. Spray lidocaine 5 times (5×10 mg) into the pharynx, repeat a second time. Hold a finger over each nostril to assess the patency of each. Spray lidocaine 10 mg $\times$ 2–3 into the most patent nostril.

- Focus the scope and note the position of the orientating v marker and the direction in which the tip of the scope can be manipulated anterior/posterior. Hold the scope as distally as possible. Lateral movement is achieved by gently twisting the scope to rotate it.

- Lubricate and warm the fibrescope or use a demist agent. Slide a tracheal tube over the scope or use a wire in the suction port as an introducer.

- Stand facing the patient and pass the scope into the left nostril at right angles to the face, along the hard palate, past the tubinates, eustachian tube, over soft palate and into pharynx. At the top of the view will be the posterior pharyngeal wall and the posterior larynx. If the scope is passed from behind the patient the view will be rotated through 180°.

- Give oxygen with a nasal catheter or a mask with an introducer port.

- Fibre-optic intubation may be assisted through a laryngeal mask or an oral mask. In small children the nipple from a baby bottle is accepted by the child. An 8 mm hole is cut obliquely into the end through which the fibre-optic scope passes. A tracheal tube can be passed over the scope and through the nipple. The nipple can then be used to stabilise the tube in the mouth or cut free.[94]

- A mask that will allow fibre-optic assisted intubation and ventilation can be made by adapting a disposable CPAP mask (Vital Signs Inc, New Jersey). The two one-way valves in the ports are removed. The port close to the nose is used for the anaesthetic circuit. One of the CPAP valves is cut to leave a cylinder. To this is attached a diaphragm of latex membrane. This diaphragm will maintain an air seal during penetration by the fibre-optic scope.[95]

Trainer

- A fibre-optic trainer can be made from a box of $35 \times 15 \times 10$ cm. Three holes are made in one end to correspond to three holes at the other. A number of partitions each with a number of holes, which are offset to imitate the position of larynx, trachea and bronchi, are fixed into the box. Negotiating the holes gives practice in manipulating the scope.[96]

Cricothyroid puncture

- Cricothyroid puncture injects a 14G or 16G IV cannula at right angles to skin. If right handed stand to the left of the patient. Keep to the mid-line by pressing thumb and index finger on either side of the trachea. Test position in the trachea by the loss of resistance to the injection of air. Aspiration of air is variable as the cannula abuts against the trachea mucosa. Pass full length of cannula into the trachea otherwise it will kink.[97–99]

- Attached to a length of green oxygen tubing and an oxygen source at a flow rate of >20 l/min, obtained from any rotameter. A small hole is cut in the tubing which can be occluded with a finger to inflate the lungs. Take care not to create a sudden, high pressure in the trachea which can cause petecheal haemorrhages in the mucosa, a pneumothorax or back flow of air through the puncture site into the neck and surgical emphysema. In children do not inflate, which will cause barotrauma, use passive insufflation.

- Cricothyroid puncture with a Tuohy needle allows an epidural catheter to be passed through the larynx to act as an introducer for a tracheal tube. If right handed stand to the right of the patient to manipulate the catheter into the mouth.

Tracheostomy

- Attachments to infant tracheostomy tubes for delivering humidified, warmed gas without disconnection or blockage are difficult to achieve. Using the Great Ormond Street (GOS) tracheostomy tube a tightly fitting tapered tube is made to fit the well of the tube with the other end fitting into the Newcastle Bridge piece. Inspiratory and expiratory tubes are fitted to the bridge piece and taken around the neck to form a collar. They are then brought forward and downward over the chest. Two pieces of adhesive tape are used to fix the tubes together as they lie at the side of the neck. The tube collar stabilises the tracheostomy tube.[100]

- A size 1 Randell Baker Soucek infant mask, with the nasal end facing caudally makes an airtight seal over a tracheostomy opening when the stoma is not cannulated. This can be used for preoxygenation, or administering a volatile anaesthetic agent[101] (Figure 6).

- An infant with a distal trachea obstruction may not be relieved by a GOS tracheostomy tube. Remedy: a 3.0 GOS tube cut at the neck, a Portex polar 3.5 mm south plain tracheal tube cut to the required length from the bend and the distal part discarded. This tube is threaded through the GOS tube. The proximal end of the polar tube is cut to level with the extension of the GOS tube and a

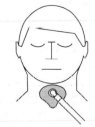

Figure 6 – Inverted mask over tracheostomy stoma.

3.5 mm tracheal tube connector fitted. This tube splints the stenosed segment and is used until a special tube can be made.[102]

Vocalisation via a cuffed tracheostomy tube

- A thin catheter is bent back on itself with holes along its length. The doubled end is passed over the upper surface of the tracheostomy tube. Air or oxygen are passed through the catheter to give a flow of gas onto the cords.[103]

Replacing a tracheostomy tube soon after a tracheostomy and before an epithelialised tract has developed can be aided by using a plain, PVC tracheal tube or suction catheter as a guide. The tube diameter should be just smaller than the internal diameter of the tracheostomy tube. The tube is well lubricated and passed to a depth of 8–10 cm into the lumen of the tracheostomy tube, which is now removed. The airway is secure and patent at all times until a new tube is in place. Oxygen is passed through catheter.[104]

Nearly healed tracheostomy

Mask ventilation or tracheal intubation and IPPV of a patient with a tracheostomy that has virtually healed may lead to air leaking through the stoma. A translucent dressing placed over the stoma will act to indicate when air is leaking. Bubbles will appear under the dressing.[105]

References

1. Chaffe A, Street MN. A modified airway. *Anaesthesia* 1988; **43:** 611.
2. Schwartz AJ, Dougal RM, Lee KW. Modification of oral airway as a bite block. *Anesthesia and Analgesia* 1980; **59:** 225.
3. Lawes EG, Murrell D. An airtight seal for bearded face. *Anaesthesia* 1985; **40:** 1142.
4. Northwood D, Wade MJ. Novel use of the Randel-Baker Soucek mask. *Anaesthesia* 1991; **46:** 319.
5. Edmondosn WC, Rushton A. The upside down face mask again. *Anaesthesia* 1992; **47:** 361.
6. Langer RA. Simple modification of a medium concentration oxygen mask improves patient comfort and respiratory monitoring with capnography. *Anesthesia and Analgesia* 1996; **83:** 202.
7. Leadbeater MJ, Nott MR. Half a guard is better. *Anaesthesia* 1990; **45:** 343.
8. Lisman R, Shepherd NJ, Rosenberg M. A modified laryngoscope blade for dental protection. *Anesthesiology* 1981; **55:** 190.
9. Haddy S. Protecting teeth during endotracheal intubation. *Anesthesiology* 1989; **71:** 810–11.
10. Singhal SK, Chhabra B. Loose tooth: a problem. *Anesthesia and Analgesia* 1996; **83:** 1352.
11. Cobley M, Dunne J. Is the pre-operative removal of dentures necessary? *Anaesthesia* 1991; **46:** 596.
12. Thomas DV. Pre-operative removal of dentures. *Anaesthesia* 1991; **49:** 1094.
13. Weller RM. Sans teeth. *Anaesthesia* 1981; **36:** 218.
14. Choi JJ. A new double-angle blade for direct laryngoscopy. *Anesthesiology* 1990; **72:** 576.
15. Skilton RWH, Parry D, Arthurs GJ, Hiles P. A study of the brightness of laryngoscope light. *Anaesthesia* 1996; **51:** 667–72.
16. Williamson R. Bimanual cricoid pressure – another version. *Anaesthesia* 1991; **46:** 510.
17. Crawford JS. The contra-lateral cuboid aid to tracheal intubation. *Anaesthesia* 1982; **37:** 345.
18. Willis B, Latto IP. Profile-cuffed tracheal tubes and the Cardiff Cuff Controller. *Anaesthesia* 1989; **44:** 524.
19. Mersch Y, Bardoczky G, d'Holland A. Tracheal tube cuff measurement – inexpensive continuous monitoring. *Anaesthesia* 1992; **47:** 1106.
20. Lineberger CK, Johnson MD. A method for preventing endotracheal tube cuff over-distention caused by nitrous oxide diffusion. *Anesthesia and Analgesia* 1991; **72:** 843–4.
21. Kim JM. The tracheal tube cuff pressure stabilizer and its clinical evaluation. *Anesthesia and Analgesia* 1980; **59:** 291–3.
22. Fisher JA, Kay J. Control of endotracheal cuff pressure using a simple device. *Anesthesiology* 1987; **66:** 253.

23. Saha AK. The estimation of the correct length of oral endotracheal tubes in adults. *Anaesthesia* 1977; **32:** 919–20.

24. Owen RL, Cheney FW. Endotracheal intubation: a preventable complication. *Anesthesiology* 1987; **67:** 255–7.

25. Tran DQ. Positioning of the endotracheal tube. *Anaesthesia and Intensive Care* 1994; **22:** 236.

26. Eagle CCP. The relationship between a person's height and appropriate endotracheal tube length. *Anaesthesia and Intensive Care* 1992; **20:** 156–60.

27. Yates AP, Harries AJ, Hatch DJ. Estimation of nasotracheal tube length in infants and children. *British Journal of Anaesthesia* 1987; **59:** 524.

28. Coldiron JS. Estimation of nasotracheal tube length in neonates. *Paediatrics* 1968; **41:** 823–8.

29. Soni AK, Paes ML. Getting the length right. *Anaesthesia* 1994; **49:** 549.

30. Bourne TM, Barker I. External diameter of paediatric tubes. *Anaesthesia* 1993; **48:** 839.

31. Levack ID, Scott DHT. Conservative management of intra-cuff puncture in a bronchial tube. *Anaesthesia* 1985; **40:** 1020–1.

32. Verborough C, Camu F. Management of cuff incompetence in an endotracheal tube. *Anesthesiology* 1987; **66:** 441.

33. Lynch M. Correct placement of tracheal tubes. *Anaesthesia* 1990; **45:** 1092.

34. Haridas RP. Condensation on tracheal tubes is commonly seen with oesophageal intubation. *British Journal of Anaesthesia* 1995; **75:** 115.

35. Muir JD, Randalls PB, Smith GB, Taylor BL. Disposable carbon dioxide detectors. *Anaesthesia* 1991; **46:** 323.

36. Zbinden S, Schupfer G. Detection of oesophageal intubation: the cola complication. *Anaesthesia* 1989; **44:** 81.

37. Pollard J. Poster. VII World Congress of Anaesthesiology, Hamburg 1980.

38. Wee MYK. The oesophageal detector device. *Anaesthesia* 1988; **43:** 27–9.

39. Pollard B. Oesophageal detector device. *Anaesthesia* 1988; **43:** 713–14.

40. Williams KN, Nunn JF. The oesophageal detector device. *Anaesthesia* 1989; **44:** 412–14.

41. Baraka A. The oesophageal detector device. *Anaesthesia* 1991; **46:** 697.

42. Haynes SR, Morton NS. Use of the oesophageal detector device in children under one year of age. *Anaesthesia* 1990; **45:** 1067–9.

43. Sood PK, Hamschmidt M, Baylis R. The esophageal detector device: Ellick's evacuator versus syringe. *Anesthesia and Analgesia* 1995; **82:** 314.

44. Horton WA, Ralston S. Cuff palpation does not differentiate oesophageal from tracheal placement of tracheal tubes. *Anaesthesia* 1988; **43:** 803–4.

45. Triner L. A simpler manoeuvre to verify proper positioning of an endotracheal tube. *Anesthesiology* 1982; **57:** 548–9.

46. Dean VS, Jurai SA. The "Roll" sign for oesophageal intubation. *Anaesthesia* 1996; **51:** 803.

47. Kalpokas M, Russell WJ. A simple technique for diagnosing oesophageal intubation. *Anaesthesia and Intensive Care* 1989; **17:** 39–43.

48. Gataure PS, Latto IP, Taylor H. Use of suction catheters as an alternative to tracheal tubes in adults. *British Journal of Anaesthesia* 1992; **69:** 657–8.

49. Madden AP. A knot for anaesthetists. *Anaesthesia* 1992; **47:** 822–3.

50. Gonzales JG. Securing an endotracheal tube. *Anesthesiology* 1988; **65:** 347.

51. Steward DJ. Fixation of reinforced silicone tracheal tubes. *Anesthesiology* 1985; **63:** 334.

52. Mathews E. Securing the endotracheal tube. *Anaesthesia* 1977; **32:** 292.

53. Young TM. Securing the endotracheal tube. *Anaesthesia* 1976; **31:** 1094–5.

54. Yamoshito M, Motokawa K. A simple method for preventing kinking of 2.5 mm I.D. endotracheal tubes. *Anesthesia and Analgesia* 1987; **66:** 800–1.

55. Shimoda O, Nakayama R, Tashiro M, Ikuta Y. A tracheal tube protector to prevent kinking. *British Journal of Anaesthesia* 1993; **70:** 326.

56. Jobes DR, Nicolson SC. An alternative method to secure an endotracheal tube in infants with mid-line facial defects. *Anesthesiology* 1986; **64:** 643–4.

57. Lewis RB. Anaesthesia for laryngoscopy: a new method of ventilation. *Anaesthesia* 1977; **32:** 366.

58. Gray DC. Temporary airway during emergency tracheostomy. *Anaesthesia* 1985; **40:** 308.

59. Mallampati SR, Gatt SP, Gugino LD, Desai SP, Waraksa B, Freiburger D, Liu PL. A clinical sign to predict difficult tracheal

intubation: a prospective study. *Canadian Anaesthetists' Society Journal* 1985; **42:** 429–34.

60. Ralston SJ, Charters P. Cuffed nasopharyngeal tube as dedicated airway in difficult intubation. *Anaesthesia* 1994; **49:** 133–6.

61. Boheimer NO, Feldman SA, Soni N. A self-retaining nasopharyngeal airway. *Anaesthesia* 1990; **45:** 72–3.

62. Mikawa K, Maekawa N, Goto R, Yaku H, Obara H. Transparent dressing is useful for the secure fixation of the endotracheal tube. *Anesthesiology* 1991; **75:** 1123–4.

63. Khorasani A, Bird DJ. Facial hair and securing the endotracheal tube: a new method. *Anesthesia and Analgesia* 1996; **83:** 886.

64. Klein DS. An endotracheal tube fixation device constructed from discarded oxygen tubing and umbilical tape. *Anesthesiology* 1984; **60:** 76.

65. Calder I, Calder J, Crockard HA. Difficult direct laryngoscopy in patients with cervical spine disease. *Anaesthesia* 1995; **50:** 756–63.

66. Savva D. Sternomental distance – a useful predictor of difficult intubation in patients with cervical spine disease. *Anaesthesia* 1996; **51:** 284–5.

67. Butler PJ. Letter. *British Journal of Anaesthesia* 1992; **69:** 225.

68. King TA, Adams AP. Predicting difficult intubation. What factors influence the thyromental distance? *Anaesthesia* 1992; **47:** 623.

69. King HK, Wamg LF, Khan AK. A modification of laryngoscopy technique. *Anesthesiology* 1986; **65:** 566.

70. Gandhi SK, Burgos L. A technique of laryngoscopy for difficult intubation. *Anesthesiology* 1986; **64:** 528–9.

71. Diaz JH, Guarisco JL, LeJeune FE. A modified tubular pharyngolaryngoscope for difficult pediatric laryngoscopy. *Anesthesiology* 1990; **73:** 357.

72. Gurmarnik S. Can traditional intubation be modified? *Anesthesiology* 1985; **63:** 464.

73. Cossham PS. Difficult intubation. *British Journal of Anaesthesia* 1985; **57:** 239.

74. Cossham PS. Gum elastic bougie and difficult tracheal intubation. *Anaesthesia* 1991; **46:** 234.

75. Cossham PS. Nasotracheal tube placement over a bougie. *Anaesthesia* 1997; **52:** 184–5.

76. Sellers WFS, Jones GW. Difficult tracheal intubation. *Anaesthesia* 1986; **41:** 93

77. Patil VU, Sopchak AM, Thomas PS. Use of a dental mirror as an aid to tracheal intubation in an infant. *Anesthesiology* 1993; **78:** 619–20.

78. Bailey AG, Knipes K, Ciraulo S. Use of the Fogarty embolectomy catheter to change a pediatric endotracheal tube. *Anesthesia and Analgesia* 1988; **67:** 1016.

79. Sizer J, Pierce JMT. Unblocking tracheal tubes. *Anaesthesia* 1992; **47:** 278–9.

80. Meakin G. A useful tip. *Anaesthesia* 1989; **44:** 535.

81. Gouverneur JM. Using an urethral catheter as a guide in difficult neonatal fibreoptic intubation. *Anesthesiology* 1987; **66:** 436.

82. Telford RJ, Searle JF, Boaden RW, Boier F. Use of a guide wire and ureteral dilator as an aid to awake fibreoptic intubation. *Anaesthesia* 1994; **49:** 691–3.

83. MacKinnon AG, Harrison AG. Nasotracheal intubation. *Anaesthesia* 1979; **34:** 911.

84. Mehta S. Nasotracheal intubation: another approach. *Anaesthesia* 1987; **42:** 1126–7.

85. Russell. Atraumatic nasal intubation. *Anaesthesia* 1996; **51:** 1084.

86. Katsnelson T et al. When the endotracheal tube will not pass over the flexible fibreoptic bronchoscope. *Anesthesia* 1992; **76:** 151.

87. Oliver JJ, Rao J. Modification of the Doughty blade for the Boyle-Davies gag. *Anaesthesia* 1994; **49:** 89.

88. Moore DC. Bloodless turbinectomy following blind nasal intubation: faulty technique? *Anesthesiology* 1990; **73:** 1057.

89. Gilbert B. An ear piece modification to facilitate nasotracheal intubation. *Anesthesia and Analgesia* 1990; **70:** 334–5.

90. Gandhi MN, Panchal ID. A simple and cheap aid to blind nasal intubation. *Anaesthesia* 1993; **48:** 173–4.

91. Cavdarski A. Inflation of the tracheal cuff as an aid to blind nasal intubation. *British Journal of Anaesthesia* 1994; **72:** 139–40.

92. Max S. More on nasotracheal intubation in children. *Anesthesiology* 1995; **83:** 1130.

93. Cox RG. Nasotracheal intubation in children. *Anesthesia and Analgesia* 1995; **82:** 1085.

94. Goskowicz R, Colt HG, Voulelis LD. Fiberoptic tracheal intubation using a nipple guide. *Anesthesiology* 1996; **85:** 1210.

95. Riley R, Coombs LJ. An inexpensive mask for fibreoptic assisted intubation. *Anaesthesia and Intensive Care* 1992; **20:** 388–9.

96. Nott MR. A trainer for fibreoptic intubation. *Anaesthesia* 1995; **50:** 570–1.

97. deLisser EA, Muravchick S. Emergency transtracheal ventilation. *Anesthesiology* 1981; **55:** 606–7.

98. Gardner MC, Pearce AC. Transtracheal ventilation. *Anaesthesia* 1996; **51:** 712.

99. Patel R. Systems for transtracheal ventilation. *Anesthesiology* 1984; **59:** 165.

100. Inkster JS, Bray RY, Maybee L. Tracheostomy tube connections for infant patients. *Anaesthesia* 1980; **35:** 595–8.

101. Aghdami A, Ellis R, Rah KH. A pediatric face mask can be a useful aid in lung ventilation on post-laryngectomy patients. *Anesthesiology* 1985; **63:** 335; Ibid. *Anaesthesia* 1991; **46:** 319.

102. Poddar S, Best CJ. Modified tracheal airway tube for distal tracheal obstruction. *Anaesthesia* 1994; **49:** 736–7.

103. Hansen A, Niemala JR, Olsen GJ. Vocalisation via a cuffed tracheostomy tube. *Anaesthesia* 1975; **30:** 78–9.

104. Richardson J, Bickford Smith P. Replacement of tracheostomy tubes. *Anaesthesia* 1988; **43:** 519.

105. Tessler MJ, Kleiman SJ. Stoma leaks and gas bubbles. *Anesthesia and Analgesia* 1992; **74:** 932–3.

Air Embolism

Detection

Suspect in any operation where large veins are exposed above the level of the heart e.g. thyroidectomy, mastectomy, head and neck surgery. Can bubbles be seen in the wound? Can froth be squeezed from the veins?

Diagnosis

- Unexplained, sudden fall in oxygenation and cardiac output.

- Doppler over root of aorta. Mill wheel murmur heard with small volume of air. Test doppler position with 1 ml air IV.

- Visible evidence of air sucked into veins.

- Gasping respiration if breathing spontaneously.

- Unexplained fall in $P_{ET}CO_2$ (this is a non-specific indicator of a fall in cardiac output). If embolism due to CO_2, P_aCO_2 will rise.

- Unexplained fall in blood pressure, bradycardia or other arrhythmia.

- Change in heart sounds (tinkling, mill wheel or gum boot). A very late sign.

Treatment

a) If blood pressure is normal:

- Pressure on wound to prevent further air entry. Occlude veins proximal to the site of air entry. Lower the operative site below the level of the heart. If possible express air bubbles through the wound.

- Flood the wound with saline.

- Give 100% oxygen. Stop N_2O.

b) If blood pressure is reduced, treatment is as above plus:

- Cardio-pulmonary resuscitation.

- If CVP line in situ try to aspirate air from right atrium.

- If all else fails, try direct aspiration from the heart through the chest wall.

Although a head down, left lateral position has been recommended, this is often impractical and of doubtful value.

Arrhythmias during Anaesthesia: Monitor the ECG

Arrhythmias are very common in everyday life. In healthy people they rarely have significance. In the presence of cardiac disease their significance is proportional to the severity of the ischaemic heart disease or left ventricular hypertrophy.

Drugs for arrhythmias:

Supraventricular – adenosine, verapamil.

Supra and ventricular – amiodarone, disopyramide, beta-blockers.

Ventricular – lidocaine. (Clinically less important: Class I: membrane stabilisers, 1A quinidine, 1B lidocaine, 1C flecainide – not used. Class II: beta-blockers, metoprolol and esmolol more beta 1 specific. Class III amiodarone, bretylium, sotalaol. Class IV calcium channel blockers, verapamil.)

If cardiac output is compromised use life support algorthims (page 44).

Abnormalities of sinus rate:

1) Sinus bradycardia <50 beats/min, exclude heart block

   • Check oxygenation and BP. Exclude *hypoxia*. Consider 100% oxygen.

   • Is patient receiving a beta-blocker?

   • Reduce inspired concentration of inhalation agent.

   • Specific therapy if causing hypotension or associated with ectopic beats: Atropine IV in 0.3 mg increments to 3 mg or increments of glycopyrronium 0.3 mg. (Complete blockade of the parasympathetic system requires atropine 80 μg/kg.)

   Heart block: epinephrine 2–10 μg/min, isoprenaline 1–10 μg/minute infusion of a dilute solution, external or transvenous pacing (see below).

2) Sinus tachycardia >140 beats/min

   • Check oxygenation. Consider 100% oxygen.

   • Check adequacy of anaesthesia, analgesia and possible awareness. Has a catecholamine been injected?

   • Ensure no CO_2 retention.

   • Check adequacy of fluid replacement.

Consider specific therapy in patients with known myocardial ischaemia, heart failure, fluid overload, thyrotoxic crisis or phaeochromocytoma.

IV beta-blocker e.g. Esmolol 40 mg over 1 min, then infusion of 4 mg/min (50–200 μg/kg/min), make a solution of 10 mg/ml in 5% dextrose or 0.9% saline. Metoprolol 1–2 mg/min, boluses up to a total of 10–15 mg.

Beware beta-blockers in patients with cardiac failure, heart block or asthma.

Heart failure: Digoxin up to 500 μg, diuretics, check potassium. Diltiazem 30 mg oral when beta-blockers contraindicated or ineffective.

Supraventricular: Adenosine IV at 2 minute intervals 3 mg, 6 mg, 12 mg (half like 5–10 s). Verapamil (calcium channel blocker) 5–10 mg IV, not if heart failure or with beta-blocker. Amiodarone 300 mg (5 mg/kg over 20–120 min, maximum 1.2 g in 24 h) slowly IV; repeat if needed (long half-life in weeks).

3) Sinus arrhythmia: Normal variation of heart beat with respiration. Lost during anaesthesia, termed loss of beat to beat or R–R variation. A possible sign of anaesthesia. No therapy.

4) Junctional bradycardia

   • Check oxygenation.

   • Ensure no hypocapnia.

   • Reduce inspired concentration of inhalation agent.

Specific therapy if causing hypotension or associated with ectopic beats: Glycopyrronium or Atropine IV 0.5 mg increments to 3 mg.

Ectopic beats

1) Atrial and junctional ectopic beats

- Check oxygenation.

- Check serum K^+. If <3.0 mmol/l, give IV infusion to a peripheral vein of K^+, maximum 40 mmol K^+ in 500 ml saline in 1 h or 0.5 mmol/kg/h. Monitor ECG.

- Consider causative agents halothane, adrenergic drugs.

- Ensure no CO_2 retention (consider IPPV in spontaneously breathing patient).

- Specific therapy if causing hypotension. Atropine or glycopyrronium IV 0.5 mg increments to 3 mg.

2) Ventricular ectopic beats (BP maintained)

- Check oxygenation.

- Ensure no CO_2 retention (consider IPPV in spontaneously breathing patient).

- Reduce causative adrenergic drugs.

- Check adequacy of anaesthesia.

- Check serum K^+. If <3.0 mmol/l, give IV infusion of K^+ (maximum 40 mmol K^+/h).

- Specific therapy if any of following present:

  a) Two ectopic beats together.

  b) R on T.

  c) Multifocal.

  d) One in ten and persistent or increasing.

  e) Causing hypotension.

First choice: Amiodarone 300 mg.

Second choice: Lidocaine 50–100 mg (1–2 mg/kg) IV bolus over 5 min. Then IV infusion 2–4 mg/min for 30 min, 2 mg/kg for 2 h, then 1 mg/kg. Maximum dose 300 mg in 30 min.

Third choice: Beta-blocker e.g. Metoprolol 1–2 mg/min (as bolus doses) up to 20 mg IV. Beware beta-blocker in patients with cardiac failure, heart block or asthma.

Paroxysmal tachycardias

1) Supraventricular tachycardia: >140 beats/min usually transient. May be atrial or junctional.

- Check oxygenation.

- Ensure no CO_2 retention (consider IPPV in spontaneously breathing patient).

- Reduce inspired concentration of volatile inhalation agent.

- Try:

  – Unilateral carotid sinus massage.

  – Diagnostic adenosine 3 mg in 1 s. At intervals of 1–2 min increasing boluses of 6 and 12 mg, up to 18 mg.

- Specify therapy if tachycardia persistent: Amiodarone, beta-blocker, calcium channel blocker Verapamil 2–5 mg IV slowly, care in patients on beta-blockers.

  – Associated with hypotension: cardiovert, start with 50 J, synchronised.

2) Ventricular tachycardia: >140 beats/min. Treatment is urgent.

- Hundred per cent oxygen.

- Institute IPPV in spontaneously breathing patient.

- Turn off volatile anaesthetic agents.

- *Specific therapy*: If pulse felt: Amiodarone 300 mg, lidocaine 50–100 mg (1–2 mg/kg) IV over 2 min; repeat up to a total of 200 mg. Then 2–4 mg/min IV infusion for 30 min, 2 mg/min for 2 h, then 1 mg/kg (maximum 300 mg/h).

  If no pulse felt or lidocaine unsuccessful: treat as ventricular fibrillation with synchronised DC shock 200 J then 360 J.

Supraventricular tachycardia and ventricular tachycardia may be impossible to differentiate. If in doubt give amiodarone or lidocaine. If potassium is low give 60 mmol KCl at 40 mmol/h.

Magnesium sulphate IV 10 ml ampoule of 50% solution contains approximately 2 mmol Mg^{++}/ml. Give 8 mmol in 10–20 min, then if necessary, 65–75 mmol over 24 h. Amiodarone 300 mg over 5–15 min or by central line 600 mg over 1 h.

Ventricular fibrillation or asystole – see cardiac arrest protocol.

Atrial fibrillation

Consider cause: thyrotoxicosis, ischaemic heart disease, hypertension, rheumatic heart disease.

Rate 100–150 beats/min. Irregularly irregular.

- Check oxygenation. Ensure no CO_2 retention.

- Specific IV therapy to control rate if associated with hypotension:

  a) Amiodarone 5 mg/kg over 20 min, repeat after 1 h with ECG monitoring.

  b) Flecainide 100–150 mg IV over 30 min.

c) Verapamil 2–5 mg. Care in patients on beta-blockers.

d) Digoxin 0.25–0.5 mg slowly. Care patients already on digoxin – check levels, low potassium.

e) Cardioversion. DC shock start 100 J.

f) Consider anticoagulation as blood can clot in atrium in 5 min.

Atrial flutter

Rate regular 130–160 beats/min with 2 : 1 or 3–4 : 1 AV block. QRS <0.12 s. Wide QRS = ventricular or supraventricular arrhythmia with bundle branch block or aberrant conduction.

- Check oxygenation. Ensure no CO_2 retention.

- Specific therapy if associated with hypotension as for atrial flutter.

Heart block

Needs ECG rhythm strip record.

1) First degree PR interval over 0.2 s.

   - Check oxygenation.

   - Reduce concentration of inhalation agent.

   - If cardiac output inadequate, epinephrine, isoprenaline or other inotrope, with a limited amount of IV fluids.

2) Second degree

   - Check oxygenation.

   - Type I – reduce concentration of inhalation agents. No specific therapy.

     Type II – likely to require pacing.

     Meanwhile: Isoprenaline infusion 0.5–1.0 µg/min. Dilute 1 mg into a large volume, 1000 ml 5% dextrose to give a solution of 1 µg/ml.

3) Third degree
- Check oxygenation.
- If ventricular rate inadequate:
  a) External pacemaker or insert IV pacemaker.
  b) Meanwhile: Isoprenaline infusion 1–10 μg/min. Dilute 5 mg in 1000 ml 5% dextrose (5 μg/ml) and titrate to give a pulse rate of 70 beats/min.

Wolff–Parkinson–White tachycardia

- Stimulate vagus.
- Disopyramide 50–150 mg IV, propranolol 1–10 mg IV, ajmaline 50–100 mg IV (very short half-life). Avoid digoxin and verapamil which may increase antegrade conduction in bundle of Hiss.
- DC cardioversion if cardiac output compromised.

Anaesthetic Machine

Safety features on anaesthetic machines

- Connection of tubing to wall: colour coded, valve specific fittings and non-interchangeable connections.
- Cylinders colour coded, pin index fitting.
- Reducing value reduces pressure to 400 kPa and maintains a constant flow while cylinder pressure falls.
- Oxygen rotameter control more prominent, knurling different, white colour coded. (Boyle was left handed otherwise UK oxygen might have been on the right hand end as in US.) Oxygen fed into back bar after nitrous oxide to reduce hypoxic mixture.
- The rotameter float turns to indicate flow. Rotation avoids sticking and errors due to static or dirt. Each rotameter is calibrated for a specific gas due to differences in viscosity affecting laminar flow in the lower tube and density affecting turbulent flow in the upper tube. The flow reading is taken from the top of the rotameter float.

- Oxygen failure alarm: driven by oxygen so sounds for limited time when oxygen pressure falls, cuts off nitrous oxide, may open circuit to air.

- Nitrous oxide flow control needle valve linked to oxygen flow control needle valve to ensure a minimum oxygen concentration of 25%.

- Carbon dioxide rotameter limited to 500 ml/min.

- Back-bar pressure relief valve opening at 34 kPa to protect apparatus.

- Patient protected from barotrauma by APL valve which opens at weight of disc plus resistance of spring (if included). Reservoir bag distends at 40–60 cmH$_2$O depending on age and make.

- Vaporisers. Filling port pin indexed and colour coded. Designed to give a constant concentration despite changes in temperature, duration of use and back pressure. High thermal capacity, mat finish to absorb heat, large wick area, temperature compensation, long connecting passage. Selectatec block and vaporiser fitting designed to prevent use of more than one vaporisers at a time (this is not a standard fitting and one bar may override another).

- Connections: 15, 22, 30 mm.

- Scavenging: reservoir to prevent excess negative pressure, high flow rate capacity to prevent back pressure. Exhaust away from air conditioning to prevent recirculation.

Oxygen

- The amount of oxygen delivered when the rotameter is turned full on is different with different machines. It is usually over 20 l/min but can be over 35 l/min, compared to 46 (range 38–53 l/min) from the emergency oxygen flush.[1,2] A case can be made for never using the emergency flush and so avoiding it becoming stuck on with the risk of awareness, when the rotameter will deliver high flows.

Checklist before using an anaesthetic machine

Gas supply
Oxygen analyser
Rotameter flow and pressure test
Oxygen failure device
Vaporisers
Scavenging
Monitors
Suction

- Connections: gas cylinders or blanking plug in place to prevent leaks (the reducing valve is not a one-way valve). Pipeline connections – tug test to ensure secure fixing. Electrical supply switched on. Suction connected. Note recent service notices and file.

- Oxygen analyser connected, switched on and recently calibrated.

- Pressure gauges. Oxygen cylinder filled with gas to 137×100 kPa at 15°C. Cylinders filled with liquid include: *nitrous oxide*, filling ratio 0.75 (weight of nitrous oxide to weight of water to fill cylinder) pressure of 40×100 kPa at 15°C, *carbon dioxide* 50×100 kPa at 15°C. Both of these gases have a density of 1.87 g/l. Amount of contents determined by weighing cylinder and subtracting the empty (tare) weight marked on the cylinder valve block. Pipeline gas supplies 400–600 kPa. Suction vacuum -66 kPa.

- Look for oxygen failure warning and bypass arrangement. Identify means for cancelling oxygen failure whistle – usually a press button.

- Start check with oxygen on and nitrous oxide off and pressure zero.

- Turn oxygen rotameter on and check it moves freely through range of scale. Use oxygen analyser to test for oxygen at common gas outlet.

- Leak test. Turn oxygen rotameter to 6 l/min and occlude common gas outlet. Bobbin should fall 5 mm as the pressure rises in the back-bar. Turn vaporiser on (particularly with TEC 4) and test again for leaks. No drop in bobbin means a leak.

- Turn oxygen supply off at cylinder and pipeline and allow system to loose pressure. Oxygen failure warning alarm should sound. Cancel by pressing button identified before starting test.

- Pressurise with nitrous oxide by turning on cylinder or pipeline. Turn on rotameter. No flow should occur until oxygen system is pressurised again. Turn on oxygen supply and repeat as for oxygen. (New machines (Standard BS 5724.2.13 1990) will not allow the nitrous oxide to flow until the oxygen is on and the pipeline is under pressure.) Turn on nitrous oxide rotameter and oxygen rotameter should turn on to give no less than 25% oxygen.

- Pressure test. Occlude common gas outlet and watch nitrous oxide rotameter drop by 5 mm to exclude leaks in back bar. Repeat with vaporiser on.

- Turn off oxygen supply and depressurise. Oxygen failure warning alarm should sound as well as cutting off the flow of nitrous oxide from the common gas outlet.

- Inspect vaporisers. Check: content indicator; ease of moving control head; back-bar seating, seals and lock on back bar; no interference with adjacent vaporiser. The vapour with the highest SVP and lowest boiling point should be placed downstream.

- Scavanging attached and turned on.

- Other monitors. Capnograph, ECG, pulse oximeter, NIBP, oxygen analyser, nerve stimulator.

See Association of Anaesthetists' checklist.

Wheels often get trapped by cables when moving a machine. Solution: A wheel cover can be made of a cylinder cut from plastic piping used in plumbing. To fit wheels of 6.5 and 12.5 cm diameter, a piece of 15 cm long piping is cut from a tubing of 16 cm diameter and 0.5 cm thick. The top and bottom edges are smoothed to slide across the floor. The covers push cables and pipes out of the way.[3]

Breathing circuits

- Visual inspection for correct assembly, deterioration in materials.

- Pressure test for leaks.

- Pressure relief valve open and close.

- Oxygen sensor in appropriate place to detect oxygen failure. Pressure alarm to detect disconnect in circuit.

1) Bain circuit

- To ensure that the central connections are airtight perform a pressure test. The central fresh gas port in the patient connector is occluded with a finger or barrel from a 2 ml syringe and, with the fresh gas flow on, the reservoir bag should not fill. When the reservoir bag has been filled

beforehand, releasing the obstruction will lead to a rapid collapse of the bag due to a venturi like effect of fresh gas, flowing from the released end, sucking gas from the outer tube.[4]

2) Lack circuit

- The outer tube can be tested by closing the exhaust valve, and with the patient end occluded no gas should be lost from a prefilled reservoir bag. To test the inner tube a tracheal tube of about 7.5 mm ID is inserted well into the inner tube at the patient end. The exhaust valve is closed and blowing down the tracheal tube should result in no movement of the reservoir bag.[5]

- An alternative way of testing the inner tube uses an obturator made from parts of BD syringes. The piston of a 10 ml syringe is cut at 3 cm from the junction with the bung to make a smaller obturator. The bung from a 20 ml syringe is fitted over the cut end to make a larger obturator.

- The outer tube is tested by placing the 20 ml bung over the distal connector of the tubing. The expiratory valve is closed and the reservoir bag inflated. Apply pressure on the reservoir bag and no leak should occur. The inner tube is tested by putting the 10 ml bung first so that both limbs are occluded. With the expiratory valve open there should be no escape of gas on pressurising the reservoir bag. If the inner limb is defective the bag will collapse and gas escapes though the expiratory valve.[6]

3) Circle

- Connect circle to common gas outlet and place a reservoir bag at the patient connector.

- Pressurise circuit by filling with gas to 40 mmHg (5 kPa) and leave for 5 min. There should be no fall in pressure.

- Detach the expiratory limb from the soda lime and occlude the tube end. No gas should flow from the soda lime if the one-way valves are closing.

Auxilliary equipment

Laryngoscope, one in use and back up for light failure. Gum elastic bougie for difficult intubation, intubating forceps, airways, tracheal tubes and connections, suction catheter. Suction with catheters. Trolley or table tilting head down. Monitors: pulse oximeter, ECG, BP, carbon dioxide, anaesthetic vapour analyser, temperature.

One-breath induction

A one-breath inhalation technique for induction of anaesthesia is pleasantly quick but needs a 4 l reservoir bag to account for the maximum vital capacity. This can be achieved by using two 2 l bags in series.[7]

Anaphylaxis and Anaphylactoid Reactions

Diagnosis of anaphylaxis: all or some of flushing and urticaria, hypoxia, oedema of face seen as a change in the contours of the lips and eyelids, reduced oxygen saturation, hypotension, increased airway pressure, bronchospasm, reduced lung compliance, laryngeal oedema.

1) Treatment. Severe reaction. Hypotension, hypoxia, oedema, bronchospasm.

- Stop causative agent.

- Epinephrine (adrenaline) 0.1–0.5 mg, dilute 1000 μg in 10 ml, and give 1–5 ml IV, repeat as needed to raise BP; 1000 μg = 1.0 ml of 1 : 1000 or 10 ml of 1 : 10,000 (1 : 1000 = 1 g in 1000 ml). The dose of epinephrine should be weight related 10 μg/kg but reduced in patients with cardiac disease.

- If hypotension is less severe choose a lower dose of adrenaline 10–100 μg.

- Oxygen by face mask, preferably a mask specific for 100% or 20 l/min, given by opening rotameter fully open.

- IV crystalloid, saline or Hartman's (not dextrose which only adds water), 1 l rapidly, use pressure bag, may need 3–10 l. A colloid may be the causative agent, only small ions are being lost, and larger molecules may cross and stay in the alveolar space reducing oxygenation.

- Establish ECG and urine output, possibly CVP monitoring but do not waste time.

2) Bronchospasm alone. Consider aspiration, pneumothorax, pulmonary oedema.

- Oxygen 100%.

- Epinephrine 100–500 μg or salbutamol 250–500 μg IV or through the tracheal tube.

3) Flushing and urticaria. If alone – due to displacement of histamine from mast cells by any drug – not allergy.

- Antihistamine H_1 antagonist chlorpheniramine 10–20 mg IV.

- Consider H_2 antagonist.

4) Secondary therapy

- Corticosteroids – hydrocortisone 100–300 mg IV.

- Infusion of epinephrine 4–8 μg/min.

- Norepinephrine (noradrenaline) 4–8 μg/min.

- Severe acidosis bicarbonate 0.5–1.0 mmol/kg, that is 0.5–1.0 ml/kg of 8.4% solution of sodium bicarbonate.

Once the patient's life is not at risk monitor urine output and consider establishing a causative agent.

Collect blood samples: 10 ml in EDTA (pink haematology tube) as soon as possible at 10 min, then 20 min, 1, 2, 6 and 24 h. Analyse for WBC (total and differential), platelets, haemoglobin and tryptase. Tryptase is a neutral protease from human mast cells and is markedly elevated in anaphylaxis. Analysis of a blood sample taken early on in any suspected anaphylactic reaction aids diagnosis.[8] Spin off the plasma and store at −20°C until despatch, together with a full case history, to nearest specialist. NARCOS provides a 24 h advisory service (0114 243 4343).

Later skin testing and information to the patient of agent(s) to avoid in the future.

Anticoagulation

DVT prophylaxis

- Once daily, subcutaneous, low molecular weight, heparin 2000–3500 units, depending on product.

- Every 8–12 h subcutaneous, heparin 5000 units

- Consider performing local blocks and putting in or taking out catheters before giving a dose of DVT prophylaxis, rather than just after.

Treatment of DVT. Start heparin IV to give APTT of 2–4 min (normal 30–40 s). Then aim for INR 2–3 with warfarin.

When warafrin is stopped an INR ratio of 1.5 is considered safe for surgery and possibly regional blocks.

Heart valve patients

- Patients with a prosthetic valve should have an INR of 3–4.

- INR <2 increases the risk of emboli and thrombus formation particularly with mitral valves.

- Warfarin should be stopped 48 h preoperatively and heparin given, by infusion not boluses, to an APTT of 60–80 s (normal 35–40 s).

- Infuse heparin by pump, 1000–2000 units/h diluted in 5% dextrose or 0.9% saline. Stop infusion 4–6 h before the operation and start again as soon as possible after the operation. Restart warfarin and stop heparin at INR of >2.

Arterial Cannulation

Assess patency of palmar arch with a pulse oximeter

- A pulse oximeter probe is placed on any finger.

- At the wrist the radial artery lies lateral to flexor carpi radialis, the ulnar artery lies lateral to flexor carpi ulnaris.

- Radial and ulnar arteries are occluded until no pulsation is detected by the oximeter. The ulnar artery is then released and the time to return of a pulsation is measured. Similarly the radial artery is released first and so a collateral flow from either side tested. The use of the pulse oximeter can be applied in every case, particularly when a patient is unable to co-operate with a modified Allen's test.[9–11]

- Consider a regular test of blood flow when a cannula is left in situ for several days in critical care areas. The pulse oximeter can detect pulsatile flows down to 4–8% of normal. No saturation or plethysmography reading will occur when there is very poor or lack of blood flow.[12]

Cannulation

- When the radial artery is difficult to locate by palpation such as in obese or hypotensive patients it can be cannulated by relying on its constant position, lying in a groove in the forearm created by the apposition of the tendons of brachioradialis and flexor carpi radialis muscles.

- The direction of the groove and artery is a straight line in the distal forearm.

- Once the groove has been located, by palpating for the tendons of these two muscles at about 4 fingers breadth below the palmar crease, the artery can be cannulated by visualising its position.[13]

- The posterior tibial artery is superficial and easily palpable posterior to the medial malleolus. It is covered by skin, subcutaneous tissue and the flexor retinaculum. To aid cannulation the foot is dorsiflexed to 90° and laterally rotated with the knee partially flexed.[14]

To reduce spillage of blood during cannulation

- Attach the barrel of a 10 or 5 ml syringe to the cannula and watch the blood flow into the cannula and syringe and not over the patient or floor[15] (Figure 7).

- Transfix the radial artery with a 19G cannula. Once the artery has been transfixed the needle is withdrawn and a 15 cm length of PVC tubing containing heparinised saline, a three-way tap and 10 ml syringe, are attached to the cannula which is slowly withdrawn and a flash back seen in the tubing. The syringe is used to

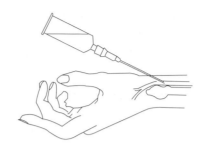

Figure 7 – Syringe barrel attached to arterial cannula to reduce blood spillage.

collect any excess fluid and to flush the cannula once in place. There is little evidence that transfixation is any more traumatic than direct cannulation.[16]

Aspiration of Vomit

Aspiration of fluid causes a sterile pneumonitis, loss of alveolar membrane integrity, pulmonary oedema and airway obstruction with solid particles.

- Place patient in head down position and on side. It is easier to intubate with the patient on their right side.

- Laryngoscopy and suction (consider bronchoscopy if solid matter inhaled).

- Proceed to intubate with a cuffed tube if patient already paralysed or there is a significant amount of aspiration. Otherwise consider waking patient.

- Suction via tracheal tube in head down position. Test aspirate with pH paper. If acid this confirms gastric aspiration. It is said that a pH below 2.5 is most damaging but there is little evidence to support this.

- Intermittent positive pressure ventilation with at least 50% oxygen, and PEEP for pulmonary oedema.

- If bronchospasm, treat with epinephrine 0.25–0.5 mg IV, or salbutamol 200 μg IV slowly.

- Methylprednisolone 2 g IV slowly (more than one dose of doubtful value).

- As necessary: blood gases, colloid for hypotension.

- Proceed with surgery if essential and patient's condition permits.

- Pass nasogastric tube and aspirate stomach.

- Chest X ray.

- Chest physiotherapy.

- Transfer to ITU care for observation of lung damage and assess need for elective IPPV.

- Antibiotics later for secondary infection.

References

1. Venn PJH. Pre-oxygenation – how long? *Anaesthesia* 1983; **38:** 703.
2. Goddard RH, Sellers WFS. Maximum oxygen flows from a Boyle's machine. *Anaesthesia* 1984; **39:** 199.
3. Sakai T, McIntyre JWR, Baba S, Matsuki A. Push and pull: move your anaesthetic machine more easily. *Anesthesia and Analgesia* 1994; **79:** 196–7.
4. Strong TS, Barrowcliffe MP. Pressure testing the anaesthetic machine and breathing system. *Anaesthesia* 1996; **51:** 88.
5. Furst B, Laffey DA. An alternative test for the lack system. *Anaesthesia* 1984; **39:** 834.
6. Martin LVH. An alternative test for the Lack system. *Anaesthesia* 1985; **40:** 80–1.
7. Lee JJ. Single breath induction of anaesthesia. *Anaesthesia* 1990; **45:** 491.
8. Fisher M. Tryptase in anaphylaxis. *Anaesthesia and Intensive Care* 1990;**19:** 479.
9. Nowak GS, Moorthy SS, McNiece WL. Use of pulse oximetry for assessment of collateral aterial flow. *Anesthesiology* 1986; **64:** 527.
10. Rozenberg B, Rosenberg M, Birkhan J. Allen's test performed by pulse oximeter. *Anaesthesia* 1988; **43:** 515–16.
11. Person E. The pulse oximeter and Allen's test. *Anaesthesia* 1992; **47:** 451.
12. Munro, FJ, Broome I. Radial artery occlusion detected by pulse oximetry. *Anaesthesia* 1994; **49:** 102.
13. Lanier WJ. An alternative technique for locating the radial artery. *Anesthesia and Analgesia* 1993; **77:** 1082–3.
14. Madan R et al. Cannulation of the posterior tibial artery. *Anaesthesia* 1990; **45:** 589–90.
15. Sabo B, Smith RB. A tidy adjunct to arterial cannulation. *Anesthesiology* 1986; **64:** 534–5.
16. Lyon MT, Armstrong A. A new technique for insertion of an intra-arterial cannula. *Anaesthesia and Intensive Care* 1990; **18:** 579–80.

Bags as Wedges

An empty intravenous bag connected to the inflating balloon from a sphygmomanometer cuff and part inflated makes a variable size wedge. Check for latex allergy.

A 1 l bag

- under the neck and shoulders or at the side of the face will conform to any shape, stabilise the head and support a breathing circuit; the plastic is not toxic to the skin;[1,2]

- under the head before thyroidectomy it is inflated to extend the neck at the beginning of surgery and deflated at the end for wound closure;

- placed under the heel, reduces pressure on the skin and calf.[3]

A 1 or 3 l bag acts as an inflatable wedge at caesarean section. A bag under each side allows a quick change in tilt if hypotension develops on one side.[4-6]

Blood and Fluid Loss

Acute blood loss in young, fit patient:

- 500 ml (10%) loss – vasoconstriction, slight increase in heart rate, no BP change, compensation by fluid shift from ECF over 1–2 h;

- 1000 ml (20%) loss – vasoconstriction, increased heart rate and respiratory rate, reduced urine output, little BP change;

- 2000 ml (40%) loss – lower blood pressure due to increased heart rate and vasoconstriction failing to maintain cardiac output;

- very fit patients can increase their cardiac output by doubling stroke volume (70–140 ml) and trebling heart rate (50–150). Any reduction in either will lead towards a fixed cardiac output and limited ability to compensate for blood loss or vasodilatation;

- elderly suffer a fall in blood pressure earlier as they are less able to compensate with vasoconstriction and tachycardia.

Preoperative anaemia[7]

Blood transfusion is rarely indicated when the haemoglobin is >9 g/dl, and usually indicated when <6 g/dl. At 10 g/dl, 660 ml oxygen/min will be delivered to the tissues with a 5 l cardiac output. At 6 g/dl, 400 ml oxygen/min will be delivered. This is not enough to extract the basal oxygen requirement of 250 ml without increasing heart rate and/or stroke volume. The decision to transfuse depends on oxygen requirement and delivery, cardiac and lung function, availability of safe blood, side effects of transfused blood and the patient's wishes. Circulating blood volume must be maintained with a suitable fluid. A patient with a low Hb may also have a low serum osmolarity leading to oedema.

Massive blood transfusion[8]

The infusion of more than 10% blood volume in 10 min (adult 500 ml) or whole body blood volume 70 ml/kg in 6 h may lead to impaired oxygenation and RDS, coagulation disorders, hypothermia, acidosis, hyperkalaemia, hypocalcaemia.

Management

- One hundred per cent oxygen.

- Two large bore 14G IV cannulae or interosseous needle.

- Two litres saline followed by 1 l of colloid.

- O negative blood if blood pressure <90 systolic in pregnancy, otherwise group specific blood.

- Once the total blood volume has been replaced it is unlikely that antibodies will exist to be detected by blood cross match. Group specific blood should be given.

- After 6 units of blood and if further rapid transfusion is likely, send blood sample for clotting screen (prothrombin time (PT) and activate partial thromboplastin time (APTT)) haemoglobin and platelets and give two or more bags of fresh frozen plasma (FFP). If FFP fails to raise the fibrinogen above 1 g/l then cryoprecipitate should be considered.

- Further FFP should be given according to results of clotting screen and clinical situation. Repeat clotting screen, as necessary.

- Fibrinogen falls to the critical level of 1 g/l after 150% blood loss. Once the PT or APTT are prolonged to 1.5 times the normal there is an increased risk of clinical coagulopathy.

- Platelets may fall to 50×10^9/l when two blood volumes have been replaced. If bleeding continues after acute replacement of half the blood volume, consider ordering 6 units of concentrated platelets (will probably be given after 10 or more units of blood).

- When using plasma reduced red cells, or red cells with optimal additive (SAG-M blood), for every 2 units of blood give 500 ml of synthetic colloid (e.g. gelatin solutions). If more than blood volume replacement use human albumen solution (HAS), if available. Every fourth unit give FFP for protein and coagulation factors.

- Check acid–base state when possible. If base deficit greater than 10 mmol/l and pH <7.2, consider cause and give 50 mmol 8.4% HCO_3.

- Calcium in haemaccel may cause precipitation if mixed with citrated blood.

- In patients with liver disease start with clotting screen, haemoglobin and platelets when initiating transfusion.

- Warm patient and all fluids.

- Monitor: urine output, ECG, arterial blood gases and electrolytes.

Acute loss: haematocrit may not be a reliable assessment of total body haemoglobin due to dilution effects.

Chronic loss: to calculate the amount of blood to be transfused:

- Assuming a circulating blood volume of 100 ml/kg, plasma reduced blood PCV 70%, whole blood PCV 40%.

- Plasma reduced blood (ml) required = desired change in haematocrit × body weight (kg) × 1.5.

- Whole blood (ml) = desired change in haematocrit × body weight (kg) × 2.5.

If circulating blood volume is 70 ml/kg:

- Plasma reduced blood (ml) = desired change in haematocrit × weight (kg) × 1.0 ml.

- Whole blood required (ml) = desired change in haematocrit × weight (kg) × 1.75.[9]

- Adequate transfusion when patient cooperative and not confused, urine output >30 ml/h and serum osmolarity >300 mosmol/l, warm periphery, no tachycardia, blood pressure over 100 systolic, depending on age and normal blood pressure.

Early consultation with a haematologist will ensure rational management of massive transfusion.

Blood replacement

ABO blood groups in population: O, 44%; A, 45%; B, 8%; AB, 3%. Group A has

A antigen and anti B antibodies in the circulation. The antigens are present in body cells and tissue fluids. The antibodies are glycoproteins with different terminal sugars and cause intravascular haemolysis. Rh antibodies are only present in Rh negative patients after exposure to Rh positive red cells. This may occur with blood transfusion or by a Rh positive baby's blood entering the circulation of a Rh negative mother.

Choice of blood for replacement:

- O negative blood in a life threatening emergency. The A and B antibodies in the transfused blood will be diluted in the recipient to give minimal reaction. Other systems are not considered but may give a reaction.

- Group specific blood. Blood of the patient's ABO Rh group is released rapidly from a blood bank. The antibody profile is better than for O negative. A cross-match test should be available in 20 min to guide further transfusion.

- Grouped blood for ABO. The slide test picks up agglutination due to other antibodies. A provisional result can be available in 20 min.

Blood with oxygen carrying capacity:

- Whole blood: 450 ml from donor with 63 ml glucose, adenine and citrate to bind calcium. Should be filtered to eliminate debris from lysed cells and fibrin.

- Packed cells: whole blood with 20–30% of the plasma removed, PCV 70%.

- SAGM or red cell concentrate blood with all the plasma removed. Red cells suspended in 100 ml saline, adenine and mannitol. The mannitol gives the fluid an osmotic pressure to prevent water entering the RBC causing swelling and lysis. PCV 65%. After 2–4 units saline, protein and then clotting factors should be added.

Clotting factors

- FFP contains all clotting factors. Prepared by freezing the 200 ml of plasma from 1 unit of donor blood.

- Platelet concentrates prepared by centrifuging pooled whole blood or plateletpheresis of a single donor. Used when platelets $<50 \times 10^9/l$.

- Cryoprecipitate: 20 ml of supernatant from FFP contains factors VIII and fibrinogen.

- Factors VIII and IX from pooled plasma; being replaced by genetically engineered factors.

Haemostatics

- Tranexamic acid inhibits plasminogen activation and fibrinolysis. Use: prostate and dental bleeding. Dose: 0.5–1 g slowly IV.

- Ethamsylate reduces capillary bleeding by platelet effect. Dose: 125–250 mg.

- Aprotinin inhibits proteolytic enzymes, inactivates kallikrein. Use: cardiac surgery (hypersensitive reaction if previous exposure).

- DDAVP 0.3 µg/kg IV over 20 min reduces the bleeding time in haemophilia and normal people. Used to reduce intraoperative bleeding during cardiac and orthopaedic operations.[10]

Measuring blood loss

- When it is important to measure small volumes of blood loss, a Buretrol or similar measuring cylinder can be placed inside the suction bottle. All the fluid drawn through the suction tubing is directed into this calibrated tube before overflowing into the larger bottle[11] (Figure 8).

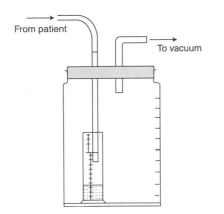

From patient

To vacuum

Figure 8 – Burette to measure blood loss from children.

Fluids and electrolytes

Kidney function

1. Eliminates the waste products of metabolism and water. Reduced renal function leads to a reduced concentrating capacity seen as nocturnia and falling urinary osmolarity.

The most important waste products that cannot be converted to carbon dioxide are potassium and some acids, either of which, in excess, will lead to death.

> Serum creatinine levels are used to assess renal function, assuming that muscle release of creatinine is constant. The elderly have a lower muscle bulk and so less creatinine is released. A raised creatinine is more significant in the elderly than in the young.

Treatment for high potassium: Calcium ions 10 mmol IV; infusion of insulin 20 units in 500 ml 10% glucose over 2 h with serum glucose monitoring; calcium resonium ion 30 g rectally or 15 g orally; 50 mmol sodium bicarbonate; dialysis.

Treatment of acidosis due to renal failure: Sodium bicarbonate to correct base deficit.

Base deficit × weight/2 = ml of 8.4% sodium bicarbonate to be given; dialysis.

2. Salt and water balance: Serum osmolarity 300 mosmol/l calculated by adding all the cations and anions (or double cations), add for glucose and urea. Healthy adults can concentrate their urine up to 4 times serum osmolarity. If the kidney is in tubular failure a glomerular filtrate will be passed with the same osmolarity as the serum. Neonates and small children have limited concentrating capacity and hence require more water for a solute load.

3. To produce hormones, renin, erythropoietin, prostaglandins.

4. Metabolism of some proteins and vitamin D.

Urine volume

Hourly measurement of urine volume indicates changes in renal blood flow and perfusion pressure. Osmolarity is a simple indicator of renal concentrating function.

Urine output in very small patients

The rubber stopper of a sterile vacutainer test tube is punctured with a Tuohy needle and one end of an epidural catheter is introduced into the tube. The Tuohy needle is discarded. A feeding tube is passed into the child's bladder and connected to the epidural catheter with a male–male connector. The length of the system is over 100 cm but the volume is less than 1 ml and urine flow will be by capillary action.[12]

Water

A 70 kg man has 45 l (2/3) water, of which 30 l (2/3) is intracellular and 15 l (1/3) extracellular. The extracellular space is subdivided into 3 l intravascular and 12 l extravascular.

33

Blood and Fluid Loss

B

A gain of 2 l (15% of ECF) will lead to oedema. A loss of 3.5 l (25% of ECF or 5% body weight) will lead to reduced skin elasticity, thirst and dry mouth. A loss of 7 l (50% ECF or 10% body weight) leads to skin turgor, low urine output, poor peripheral perfusion and hypotension.

Fluids for replacement

Crystalloids

- Saline and Hartman's solutions distribute according to the intravascular to extravascular volume ratio of about 3 : 12. If 1 l is infused, 800 ml will quickly pass into the extravascular space. One litre of either contains the adult daily requirement for sodium chloride.

- Dextrose is equivalent to giving water and will only transiently fill the intravascular space. Five per cent contains 50 g dextrose per 1000 ml or 200 cal.

Colloids

1. Gelatines: mean molecular weight 35,000, but no charge, half-life 3 h depending on renal excretion. Cheap, no effect on circulating clotting factors.

   - Gelofusin – succinylated gelatine in normal saline solution.

   - Haemaccel – urea linked gelatine; 6.26 mmol/l calcium will clot transfused blood, if in the same IV line, contains 5.1 mmol/l K^+.

2. Etherified starch: hetastarch mean molecular weight 450,000. Pentastarch mean molecular weight 200,000 to 250,000; half-life 6 h. Expands circulation, effect for 24 h, taken up by reticular endothelium. Plasma substitutes of choice when capillary leak is occurring.

3. Dextran: polysaccharides mean molecular weight 40, 70 and 110 × 1000. Can cause anaphylactic reaction; interferes with blood cross match; prophylaxis for DVT and 40 improves peripheral blood flow.

Blood products

- Whole blood: problems: cross match, infections, cold, acid, high potassium, low calcium, debris and particles from cell membranes, immunosupression.

- SAGM blood: red cells 150–250 ml suspended in 100 ml 0.9% saline with adenine 1.25 mmol/l, mannitol 20 mmol/l to maintain tonicity in place of plasma proteins and anhydrous glucose 45.5 mmol/l. PCV 60%.

- Plasma protein solutions, albumin, FFP, platelets. To replace specific losses e.g. colloid pressure, clotting factors.

Daily requirements

Water
1. Neonate:

   - Day 1, 20 ml/kg; day 2, 40 ml/kg and increasing by 20 ml/kg/day until end of first week, then 150 ml/kg/day.

2. Child after first week of life:

   - 0–10 kg; 100 ml/kg/day.

   - 10–20 kg; 1000 ml + 50 ml/kg/day.

   - 20–30 kg; 1500 ml + 30 ml/kg/day.

3. Adult: 30 ml/kg.

Electrolytes
- Sodium chloride: 2 mmol/kg/day.

- Potassium: 1 mmol/kg/day.

Thousand ml of 0.9% saline contains 154 mmol of sodium, Hartman's 1000 ml contains 140 mmol. Both contain a normal daily requirement of sodium but need to add potassium 1 mmol/kg/day.

Postoperative regime

Basic requirements for an adult: 1000 ml 0.9% saline or 1000 ml Hartman's plus 1000–2000 ml 5% dextrose. Add potassium 40–80 mmol/day to one of the bags.

Children: 0.18% saline in 4% dextrose or half-strength saline in dextrose, volumes see above.

Intravenous fluid can be prevented from back flowing into the IV line if a blood pressure reading is to be taken from the same arm by running the IV line under the cuff close to the air bladder, close the Velcro over the tubing.[13]

The most effective way of increasing the rate of flow of IV fluid is by using a 300 mmHg pressure bag with automatic adjustable pressure regulator. This can double the rate of flow. A 14G cannula rather than a 16G cannula increases flow by 50%. Manual compression of the drip chamber, even to a pressure of 100 cmH$_2$O is inefficient.[14]

Sodium

Sodium normal 135–145 mmol/l
        low <130 mmol/l.

Causes of low serum sodium

1. *Elderly*: effect of a sodium losing diuretic is to pass more urine, feel thirsty, drink water, dilute serum electrolytes. This effect may be aggravated by an ACE inhibitor which blocks aldosterone function. Aldersterone would normally retain sodium but in its absence the serum sodium falls further.

2. *Pregnancy*: normal pregnancy leads to retention of water and dilution of sodium. The sodium is further diluted by dextrose infusions and oxytocic drugs. The administration of oxytocic agents to induce labour or abortion has an antidiuretic effect.

3. *TURP syndrome*: absorption of water from the prostatic capillary bed dilutes the serum sodium.

Treatment

One hundred percent oxygen, IPPV.

Hypertonic saline 1.8%, 4.5%, 5%.

Fitting occurs below 120 mmol Na$^+$ or a sudden fall to 125 mmol.

Potassium

*   A serum potassium of above 3.5 mmol/l is desirable before elective surgery; 3.0–3.5 mmol/l is acceptable for emergency surgery if it is corrected soon. Patients with chronic hypokalaemia having operations rarely exhibit intraoperative dysrrhythmias. Symptomatic preoperative dysrhythmias are a stronger predictor of intraoperative dysrhythmias. It is possible to safely anaesthetise patients with a serum potassium of 2 mmol/l although less than 2.7 mmol/l should be considered an additional risk.[15]

*   A recommended maximum infusion of potassium for an adult is 10–20 mmol/h or 500 mmol/24 h.[16] This rate is probably conservative when the rate of redistribution from blood into the cells is taken into account[17] and 0.5 mmol/kg/h is an alternative regime. Maintenance doses of potassium are 3–4 mmol/h or 80 mmol/24 h.[18]

Resuscitation with no IV equipment

A 20 kg boy had been drifting in a boat for 10–14 days and was severely dehydrated; 70 ml/kg of warm water to which was added about 15 g table salt and about 100 g sugar were administered through a rectal tube as there was no IV equipment available.[19]

Acid–base balance

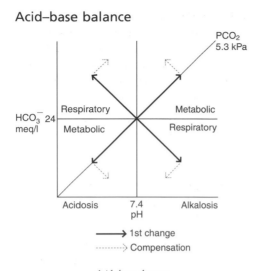

Acid–base changes.

Metabolic acidosis

In diabetes acidosis there is a lack of insulin and high glucagon. This leads to a low malonyl CoA which allows fatty acids to enter the mitochondria. The fatty acids are oxidised to acetyl CoA in too large an amount to enter the Krebs (TCA) cycle. Acetyl CoA cannot reconvert to fatty acid which requires insulin so it forms the ketoacids acetone, beta OH butyric acid and acetoacetic acid.

Treatment

See diabetes – rehydration, insulin 3–4 units/h reducing to 1–2 units/h, potassium 10 mmol in dextrose saline solution 1000 ml/4 h. Monitor urine output, serum electrolytes and glucose until stable. A similar problem exists in starvation when excess fatty acid is metabolised without carbohydrate.

Hypoxia causes a lactic acidosis. Oxygen is required for the Krebs cycle. In hypoxia the cycle slows, pyruvate from CHO metabolism cannot enter and so converts to lactic acid.

Features

Low pH, low HCO_3, compensated low CO_2. Lactic acid is increased in hypoxic states, exercise and starvation.

Metabolic alkalosis

Vomiting of gastric HCl leads to dehydration with low plasma chloride and compensatory rise in bicarbonate ion. Low plasma sodium and pottassium due to the kidney retaining hydrogen ions. Symptoms include dehydration, confusion and neuromuscular irritability.

First correct the hypovolaemia, hyponatraemia and hyokalaemia with solutions containing sodium chloride and potassium IV or exceptionally an enema. If the chloride ion remains low consider an enema of 200 ml calcium chloride. Leave in place for 3 h and repeat as necessary after 12 h. Calcium chloride is used as calcium is only absorbed by the ileum.[20] Sodium and potassium are absorbed by the colonic wall.

What is pH?

pH = negative $\log_{10}$ hydrogen ion concentration. If hydrogen ion concentration is 50 neq/l $= 50 \times 10^{-9}$ or 5×10^{-8}; log 5 is about $+0.7$ and log 10^{-8} is -8. These are now added to give -7.3, but pH is negative log so pH $= 7.3$

Changing pH to H^+ (between values of pH 7.10 and 7.60.)[21–25]

• The sum of the hydrogen ion concentration in nmol/l and the numerical value of the two digits after the decimal point of the pH number is relatively fixed around 80 (83 is a more exact number).

• To convert H^+ to pH, subtract the H^+ concentration from 80 to give the two digits after 7 and the decimal point.

• To convert pH to H^+ the two number value after the decimal point is subtracted from 80.

Blood Pressure

- The cuff should not act as tourniquet. The width of the cuff should be the diameter of the arm + 20% or half the circumference.

- The reading of blood pressure varies with position. In the lateral position systolic and diastolic blood pressure readings are over 10 mmHg lower than in the supine position.[26]

- The blood pressure in patients with hemipareses should be measured in the non-paralysed arm to avoid errors by measuring from the paralysed arm.[27] The pressure in the paralysed limb may be higher or lower than the actual pressure.

- The pulse is usually lost to palpation at 50–60 mmHg. Accurate measurement of blood pressure in infants and hypotensive patients can be obtained using an ultrasound flow detector. Low flows can be detected by placing the probe over a peripheral pulse and connecting to an auditory output.[28]

Brainstem Death

Criteria for assessing brainstem death:

- Patient has brain damage of known aetiology.

- There is no drug effect e.g. narcotic, hypnotic, tranquilliser, alcohol.

- No hypothermia affecting brain function.

- Circulatory, metabolic and endocrine causes for reduced consciousness are excluded.

- The patient is ventilated for apnoea not caused by drugs such as muscle relaxants.

All brainstem reflexes must be absent.

- Pupils fixed and non-responsive to a sharp change in the intensity of incidental light.

- No corneal reflexes.

- No vestibulo-ocular reflexes. No eye movement during the slow injection of 50 ml ice water over 1 min into each external auditory meatus. Inspect for wax, head up 30°. It may not be possible to use both ears due to trauma.

- No motor response within the cranial nerve distribution.

- No limb movement to supraorbital pressure.

- No gag reflex or reflex response to bronchial stimulation by suction catheter in tracheal tube.

- No respiratory movement while disconnected from the ventilator. The $PaCO_2$ should reach 6.65 kPa, a level to stimulate respiration. Measured by arterial blood gases. Before the test prevent hypoxia by ventilating with 100% oxygen for 10 min then with 5% carbon dioxide for 5 min. Then discontinue ventilation for the test with oxygen flowing through a catheter in the trachea.

Children over 2 years are treated as adults. Below 2 years it is rarely possible to diagnose brain stem death with confidence.

The tests are performed by two doctors together or separately, who are competent in the field, not members of the transplant team and registered for at least 5 years. At least one must be a consultant. Two sets of tests are necessary. The period between each test is based on clinical judgement. The legal time of death is when the first test confirms brain stem death but death is pronounced after the second test.[29]

Bronchial Obstruction

- A blood clot or mucus plug, lodged in a bronchus, can be removed with a Fogarty or a Foley catheter. The catheter is passed through a bronchoscope and beyond the clot, the balloon is inflated and the catheter withdrawn pulling before it the clot.[30]

- Oxygen can be passed through the catheter lumen to maintain oxygenation.

Bronchial Lavage

- A 5F or 8F infant feeding catheter is attached to a syringe holding 1 ml/kg isotonic, warmed saline and a small quantity of air. The syringe should be capable of holding twice this volume. After pre-oxygenation the catheter is passed blindly until it wedges in a bronchus. The fluid is injected with a little air to clear the dead space, and then aspirated using the syringe. If no fluid is obtained the catheter is withdrawn by 1 cm and suction repeated; 30–50% of the injected volume should be returned and part sent for microbiological analysis.[31]

Bronchospasm during Anaesthesia

Treatment

- Relieve any mechanical cause.

- Hundred per cent oxygen.

- Bronchodilators.

- Salbutamol 200 μg slowly IV or through the tracheal tube. Then start infusion at 5 μg/min adjust to 3–20 μg/min IV.

- Aminophylline 250–500 mg IV slowly. Then 500 μg/kg/h, adjust to plasma theophylline concentration. Small margin between therapeutic and toxic levels.

Consider:

- Epinephrine (adrenaline) 250–500 μg.

- Isoprenaline, Halothane, Ketamine, Atropine.

- Magnesium sulphate to begin with 1–2 g (2–4 mmol Mg^+) but monitor cardiac function, blood pressure and muscle power.

- Any one or a combination of the above drugs may be effective.

- Monitoring: Pulse oximeter, ECG, Arterial gases.

- Hydrocortisone 200 mg IV, every 4 h.

Bronchospasm during anaesthesia
Differentiate from other causes of expiratory wheeze and failure to ventilate:

1. Machine
   Use self-inflating bag.

2. Airway and tube
   Tracheal tube in oesophagus or right bronchus. Kinked or partially blocked tubes. Over-distended cuff.

3. Patient
   Bronchospasm, anaphylaxis, pulmonary oedema, inhalation of FB, pneumonia, pneumothorax.
   Drugs
   – Histamine releasing drugs.
   – Non-selective B-blocker.
   – Adverse drug reaction.

An expiratory wheeze suggests a distal airway obstruction, stridor or wheeze during inspiration suggests an upper airway obstruction. A wheeze throughout the respiratory cycle suggests obstruction within the breathing equipment.

Management of acute asthma in A&E department

Consider that the patient

- may have been breathless for hours or days;

- has been self-medicating or had a precipitating cold for days;

- is exhausted, dehydrated due to hyperventilation, and retaining sputum with mucus plugs.

Paralyse and ventilate immediately (do not transfer to another ward) if exhausted (rising heart rate and respiratory rate, unable to cough, unable to talk).

- *Arterial gases*: Oxygen: oxygen tension may be artificially high due to added inspiratory oxygen. Carbon dioxide: P_aCO_2 low if hyperventilating; if P_aCO_2 is normal or above normal the patient may be so exhausted that they have stopped hyperventilating; the CO_2 is rising and they will die within minutes.

- Intubate and ventilate in order to oxygenate, control carbon dioxide, humidify airways, aspirate mucus plugs from lung and avoid collapse from exhaustion. Do not transfer to another ward if exhausted. Anaesthetise and intubate immediately wherever the patient is.

- Falling blood pressure indicates dehydration, reduced myocardial function and a low cardiac output.

Burns

To assess pecentage of skin burnt:

Table 2

	Adult rule of 9s[32]	Children rule of 10s
Head	9%	20%
Trunk front	18%	20%
Trunk back	18%	20%
Each arm	9%	10%
Each leg	18%	10%

Fluid replacement = body weight × % burn = ml crystalloid in each period reduced by 50% if colloid (plasma protein fraction).[33]

Periods (h):

1) 0–4, 2) 4–8, 3) 8–12,
4) 12–18, 5) 18–24, 6) 24–36.

- Start time of first and subsequent periods from time of burn, not time of admission.

- Alternative formula 2 ml/kg×% burn by 8 h and repeat by 16 h.[34]

- Adequacy of fluid resuscitation is judged by urine output at least 0.5 ml/kg/h.[35]

- Full thickness (i.e. loss of skin sensation) gives 50% fluid as blood.

- Inhalation injury.

- Suspect if soot in nostril, coughing, voice change, respiratory distress.

- Intubate immediately; danger from laryngeal oedema which develops rapidly.

References

1. Bembridge M. An inflatable paediatric wedge. *Anaesthesia* 1987; **42**: 213.
2. Ward ME. Eye protection during anaesthesia. *Anaesthesia* 1978; **33**: 556–7.
3. Brighouse. A simple inexpensive method to prevent heel sores. *Anesthesiology* 1986; **64**: 536.
4. Casale FF. An inflatable wedge. *Anaesthesia* 1983; **38**: 172.
5. Carrie LES. An inflatable obstetric anaesthetic wedge. *Anaesthesia* 1982; **37**: 745–7.
6. Gurmarnik S, Horowitz J. Bilateral uterine displacement device. *Anesthesiology* 1986; **64**: 654.
7. Chen AY, Carson JL. Perioperative management of anaemia. *British Journal of Anaesthesia* 1998; **81(Suppl.1)**: 20–4.
8. Stainsby D, MacLennan S, Hamilton PJ Measurement of massive blood loss: a template guideline. *British Journal of Anaesthesia* 2000; **85**: 487–91.
9. Cassady JF, Patel RI, Epstein BS. Calculations for predicting blood transfusion needs. *Anesthesiology* 1983; **59**: 491.
10. Stone DJ, DiFazio CA. DDAVP to reduce blood loss in Jehovah's witnesses. *Anesthesiology* 1988; **69**: 1028.

11. Wilkinson DJ, Redmond J. Measurement of blood loss in children. *Anaesthesia* 1994; **39:** 72.

12. Friedman–Mor Z, Nyman DJ. A simple device for monitoring urine output in very small patients. *Anesthesia and Analgesia* 1994; **79:** 605.

13. Brin EN, Lewis TC, Brin JA. A simple method for reducing backup of blood into intravenous lines caused by inflation of a blood pressure cuff. *Anesthesia and Analgesia* 1990; **71:** 569.

14. Stoneham MD. An evaluation of methods of increasing the flow rate of i.v. fluid administration. *British Journal of Anaesthesia* 1995; **75:** 361–5.

15. Wong KC, Sperry R. What is an acceptable preoperative serum potassium level for surgery? *Anesthesiology* 1994; **81:** 269.

16. Vaughan RS. Potassium in the perioperative period. *British Journal of Anaesthesia* 1991; **67:** 194–200.

17. Vickers MD. Potassium in the perioperative period. *British Journal of Anaesthesia* 1992; **68:** 224–5.

18. Potassium disorder and cardiac arrhythmia. *Drugs and Therapeutic Bulletin* 1991; **29:** 73–4.

19. Wells DG, Tredrea CR, Cooper D. An old but useful form of fluid resuscitation. *Anesthesiology* 1992; **76:** 868.

20. Evora PRB. Treatment of hypochloraemic metabolic alkalosis by rectal infusion of calcium chloride. *Critical Care Medicine* 1985; **13:** 874.

21. Walling PT. Converting pH to H$^+$. *British Journal of Anaesthesia* 1997; **79:** 262–3.

22. Burden RJ, McQuillan PJ. Converting pH and H$^+$: a rule of thumb. *British Journal of Anaesthesia* 1997; **78:** 479.

23. Serpell MG. ABGs as easy as ABCs. *Anaesthesia* 1991; **46:** 71.

24. Hope A, Farling PA. Conversion of pH to H$^+$ concentration in nmol/litre. *Anaesthesia* 1990; **45:** 699.

25. Leon-Ruiz EN. A simple way to convert pH to hydrogen ion concentration. *Anesthesiology* 1983; **59:** 155.

26. Meyerstein N, Chayoth R. Apparent blood pressure values in lateral recumbency. *Anaesthesia* 1982; **37:** 98–9.

27. Moorthy SS et al. Blood pressure monitoring in hemiplegic patients. *Anesthesia and Analgesia* 1996; **82:** 437.

28. Thick MG, Thick GC. Monitoring low blood pressure. *Anaesthesia* 1978; **33:** 726–8.

29. Cadaveric organ transplantation. A code of practice including the diagnosis of brain death. HMSO, London 1983.

30. Smurthwaite GJ, MacDonald IJF. Another use of the Fogarty catheter. *Anaesthesia* 1995; **50:** 86.

31. Schindler MB, Cox PN. A simple method of bronchoalveolar lavage. *Anaesthesia and Intensive Care* 1994; **22:** 66–8.

32. Lund CC, Bowder NC. Estimation of area of burns. *Surgery, Gynecology and Obstetrics* 1944; **79:** 352.

33. Muir IFK, Barclay TL, Settle JAD. The practical management of burns shock. In: Burns and their Management 3rd edn. pp. 30–5. Butterworth, London.

34. Parkland formula: Deutch EA. *Burn management.* p 1507. In: Rippe JM et al. *Intensive Care Medicine*, Brown, Boston 1991.

35. Settle JAD. Urine output following severe burns. *Burns* 1974; **1:** 23–42.

Capnography

If only one monitor is allowed many anaesthetists would select a capnograph, such is the information that can be inferred from the measurement of carbon dioxide.

Information from capnograph.

Respiratory rate.

Tracheal intubation.

End tidal and hence arterial carbon dioxide tension.

Ventilation to perfusion inequalities.

Estimation of cardiac output and shows sudden changes in output.

Uses

1. Monitor breathing during sedation. Carbon dioxide measurement will be less liable to dilution with air or supplemental oxygen and the level nearer to end tidal if the sample is taken distally.

   - *Mask.* Make a slit between two or three of the vent holes. A gas sampling tube can then be passed through the slit.[1,2]

   - *Nasal catheters.* One limb is used for sampling while oxygen is given through the other limb,[3] or an IV cannula is passed through one limb of the nasal catheter into the nostril.[4]

Paediatric breathing system sampling is associated with a number of difficulties and solutions.

   - Sampling of gas from the distal tracheal tube gives the best approximation to arterial PCO_2. A Portex 8.5/6.0 mm Mini-link tracheal tube connector fits into a 8.5 mm Mini-link angled connector. An intravenous cannula with extension tubing fits into the 8.5/6.0 mm connector to act as the sampling port from within the tracheal tube.[5]

   - A manometer line is fed through the distal hole in the Jackson-Rees bag and back up to the tracheal tube.[6]

   - A catheter or 14G IV cannula is placed through the suction port on the swivel connector bung.[7]

   - An 8.5 mm stainless steel plug carrying a 1 mm sampling tube 2.5 cm long fits into the 8.5 mm angled connector with the tubing into the tracheal tube.[8]

2. Detect tracheal or oesophageal intubation:

   - Carbon dioxide can be present in the stomach either from forcing expired gas into the stomach using a face mask to ventilate before intubation or from carbonated drinks and anteacids. Both can lead to the release of carbon dioxide in the stomach. This may give a false sense of security if a qualitative CO_2 detector is used to differentiate between oesophageal and tracheal intubation.[9,10]

3. Measurement of respiratory rate. Rebreathing gives a rise in the baseline level. End-tidal concentration and arterial partial pressure of carbon dioxide.

   - Normal capnograph trace is almost a vertical rise to a plateau and a rapid descent. Just before the descent is the end-tidal alveolar gas containing the end-tidal carbon dioxide concentration which approximates to arterial carbon dioxide partial pressure (Figure 9).

   - When the rise is sloped, different concentrations of carbon dioxide are coming from alveoli with different ventilation/perfusion ratios. This is a non-specific indicator of cardiac or respiratory disease.

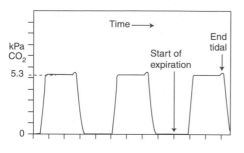

Figure 9 – Normal capnograph trace.

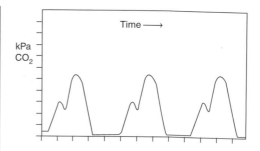

Figure 10 – Biphasic waveform with kyphoscoliosis.

4. Guide to cardiac output:

    • The area under the curve on a
      capnograph is an indication of the total
      carbon dioxide expired. A reduced
      area means a reduced volume
      eliminated. This may occur with a
      reduced lung blood flow from a
      reduced cardiac output, or rarely
      reduced carbon dioxide production as
      in hypothermia.

    • A decrease in end-tidal carbon dioxide
      concentration can indicate a reduction
      in pulmonary blood flow often several
      minutes before the changes in systemic
      haemodynamics. Acidosis should be
      corrected which may increase
      pulmonary vascular resistance and
      further decrease pulmonary blood
      flow.[11]

5. Circuit disconnection and tube kinking:

    • Sudden reduction in carbon dioxide
      concentration.

6. Different lung compliances:

    • A biphasic carbon dioxide excretion
      waveform may occur in a patient
      when the two lungs have different
      mechanics, as in kyphoscoliosis.
      Unilateral and potentially treatable,
      causes for a biphasic waveform include
      unilateral lung mass, endobronchial
      intubation and pneumohaemothorax[12]
      (Figure 10).

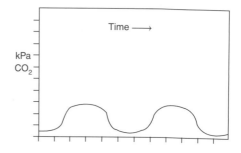

Figure 11 – Tracheoesophageal fistula.

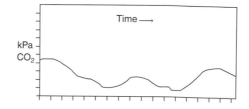

Figure 12 – Mixing of inspiritory and expiritory gases
occurs with faulty water trap of rapid respiratory rate.

7. A 1-month old was being investigated
    for gastro-oesophageal reflux. A
    particular capnograph pattern developed
    during oesophageal suction as gas was
    sucked from the trachea into the
    oesophagus indicating a
    tracheoesophageal fistula[13] (Figure 11).

8. Air entrainment:

    • An elevated inspired carbon dioxide
      and a depressed expired carbon
      dioxide can occur with a rapid
      ventilatory rate (60/min) (Figure 12);
      a long sample line; a low sample rate

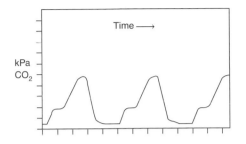

Figure 13 – Air entrapment occurs with loose sampling line connection.

(66 ml/min); a faulty water trap or other part of the analyser allowing inspired and expired gas to mix[14] (Figure 13).

- A low plateau followed by an end expiratory peak occurred due to entrainment of room air at a loose connection between the sampling line and the capnograph[15].

Some capnographs may need a software update to compensate for changes with altitude when converting from per cent to mmHg values. They over estimate values of PCO_2 when given as a per cent. This is due to the formulae PCO_2 mmHg $= FCO_2 \times$ (PB PH_2O). If a capnograph reads dry gas, $PB-PH_2O$ is calculated using PB as the atmospheric pressure and PH_2O as 0.[16]

Cardiac Arrest

The protocols produced here are those found on the UK Resuscitation Council web site www.resus.org.uk. Similar ones are published in the Journal Resuscitation vol. 46 August 23 2000, pages 1–448.

Basic Life Support

If there is a primary cardiac arrest in theatre send for help, give 100% oxygen, discontinue anaesthesia and surgery, start chest compressions, intubate and ventilate if not already doing so, ratio 15:2. Look for a cause.

Outside theatre

Follow basic and advanced life support algorithms.

Go for help first unless it is a primary respiratory arrest.

Assess ABC. The ratio of chest compression to ventilation should be 15:2 whether it is one or more people working. If the patient is intubated chest compression should continue at the same time as ventilation without a pause. A laryngeal mask airway or Combitube are alternatives to a tracheal tube. Use epinephrine 1 mg boluses IV or 2–3 mg into the tracheal tube.

Defibrillation

Use 200 J first as it causes little myocardial damage, then 200 J as the first shock reduces transthoracic impedance, then 360 J. VF consider: Amiodarone 300 mg diluted in 20 ml dextrose IV, followed by 150 mg and an infusion of 1 mg/min for 6 h to maximum of 2 g, magnesium 8 mmol if there is a deficiency. Lidocaine should not be given if amiodarone has been given but can be given alone 30 mg/min to 3 mg/kg. Procainamide is an alternative. Bretylium is not recommended. Bicarbonate may be given if the pH is <7.1 (H^+ >80 mmol/l) or if arrest is associated with a tricyclic overdose or hyperkalaemia.

Safe use of defibrillator

Switch on ECG and connect leads: red to right shoulder, yellow to left shoulder, green anywhere. Switch on defibrillator

43

but do not charge. Check ECG rhythm Lead II.

Pads to chest skin not over anything. Paddles on pads.

Stand clear, remove oxygen.

Charge to 200 J only with paddles firmly on chest.

Shock, check rhythm, repeat CPR 15 : 2 × 4.

Either re-shock or ask assistant to turn off defibrillator before taking paddles off chest. Do not wave paddles in the air.

Asystole

CPR and first dose of epinephrine 1 mg, atropine 3 mg IV or 6 mg in 10 ml into the tracheal tube.

Pulseless electrical activity

CPR and epinephrine 1 mg every 3 min, no more. Then atropine 3 mg IV or 6 mg in 10 ml to the tracheal tube.

A pregnant mother should be tilted to one side to displace the uterus off the vena cava, or the uterus displaced with the palm of the hand. The same problem can occur with any large intra-abdominal mass.

Inhaled foreign body

Adult use the Heimlick manoeuvre when a patient has inhaled a foreign body.

Child can be held upside down and slapped on the back.

Algorithms

Life support algorithms.[17]

Adult basic life support

CHECK RESPONSIVENESS	Shake and shout
OPEN AIRWAY	Head tilt/chin lift
CHECK BREATHING	Look, listen and feel
BREATHE	2 effective breaths
ASSESS 10 s only	Signs of a circulation

If breathing: recovery position

CIRCULATION PRESENT Continue rescue breathing	NO CIRCULATION Compress chest
Check circulation Every minute	100 per minute 15 : 2 ratio

Send or go for help as soon as possible according to guidelines

Advanced life support algorithm for the management of cardiac arrest in adults

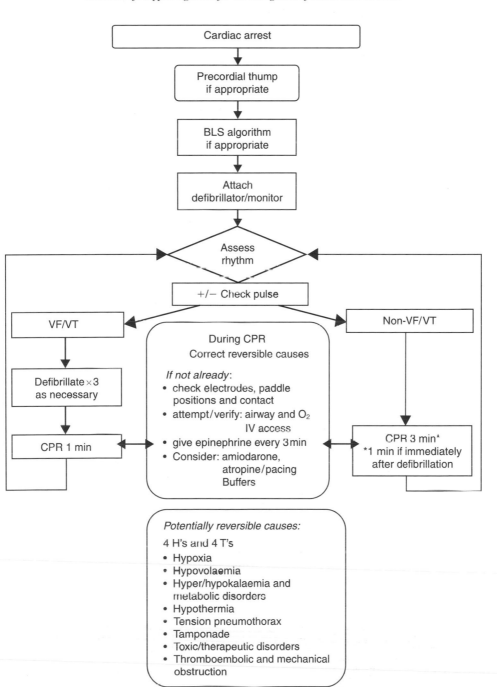

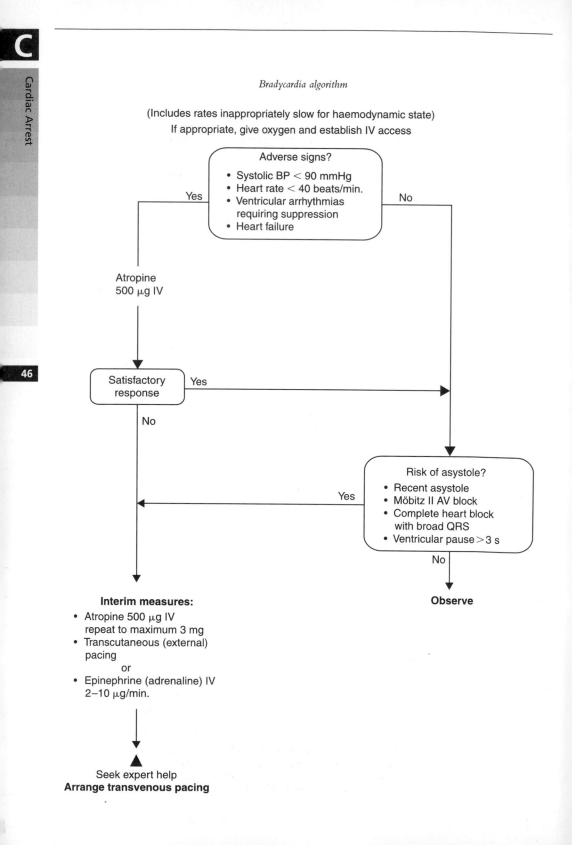

Bradycardia algorithm

(Includes rates inappropriately slow for haemodynamic state)
If appropriate, give oxygen and establish IV access

Adverse signs?
- Systolic BP < 90 mmHg
- Heart rate < 40 beats/min.
- Ventricular arrhythmias requiring suppression
- Heart failure

Yes   No

Atropine
500 μg IV

Satisfactory response — Yes

No

Risk of asystole?
- Recent asystole
- Möbitz II AV block
- Complete heart block with broad QRS
- Ventricular pause > 3 s

Yes

No

Interim measures:
- Atropine 500 μg IV repeat to maximum 3 mg
- Transcutaneous (external) pacing
        or
- Epinephrine (adrenaline) IV 2–10 μg/min.

Observe

Seek expert help
Arrange transvenous pacing

Broad complex tachycardia algorithm

(Treat as sustained ventricular tachycardia)*

If not already done, give oxygen and establish IV access

Pulse? — No → **Use VF protocol**

Yes

Adverse signs?
- Systolic BP < 90 mmHg
- Chest pain
- Heart failure
- Rate > 150 beats/min

No — Yes

Seek expert help

If potassium known to be low, *see panel*

- Give potassium chloride up to 60 mmol, maximum rate 30 mmol/hour
- Give magnesium sulphate IV 5 ml 50% in 30 min

Synchronised DC shock[†]
100 J : 200 J : 360 J
or equivalent biphasic energy

- Amiodarone 150 mg IV over 10 min,
  or
- Lidocaine IV 50 mg over 2 min repeated every 5 min to a maximum dose of 200 mg

If potassium known to be low, *see panel*

Seek expert help

- Amiodarone 150 mg IV over 10 min

Synchronised DC shock[†]
100 J : 200 J : 360 J
or appropriate biphasic energy

Further cardioversion as necessary

If necessary, further amiodarone 150 mg IV over 10 min, then 300 mg over 1 h and repeat shock

For refractory cases consider additional pharmacological agents: amiodarone, lidocaine, procainamide or sotalol; or overdrive pacing

Caution: drug induced myocardial depression

Doses throughout are based on an adult of average body weight

* Note 1: For paroxysms of torsades de pointes, use magnesium as above or overdrive pacing (expert help strongly recommended).
[†] Note 2: DC shock is always given under sedation/general anaesthesia.

Narrow complex tachycardia algorithm

(presumed supraventricular tachycardia)

| Pulseless (heart rate usually > 250 beats min⁻¹ | ◀----- | **Narrow complex tachycardia** | ----▶ | **Atrial fibrillation** |

Synchronised DC shock
100 J : 200 J : 360 J
or appropriate biphasic energy†

If not already done, give oxygen and establish IV access

Follow AF algorithm

Vagal manoeuvres
(caution if possible digitalis toxicity acute ischaemia, or presence of carotid bruit for carotid sinus massage)

Adenosine 6 mg by rapid bolus injection; if unsuccessful, follow, if necessary, with up to 3 doses each of 12 mg every 1–2 min*
Caution with adenosine in known Wolff–Parkinson–White syndrome

▲— Seek expert help

| Adverse signs? |
| • Systolic BP < 90 mmHg |
| • Chest pain |
| • Heart failure |
| • Heart rate > 200 beats/min |

No

Yes

Choose from:

• Esmolol: 40 mg over 1 min + infusion 4 mg/min
  (i.v. injection can be repeated and infusion increased incrementally to 12 mg/min

or

• Verapamil 5–10 mg IV **

or

• Amiodarone: 300 mg IV over 1 h, may be repeated once if necessary

or

• Digoxin: maximum dose 500 μg IV over 30 min × 2

Synchronised DC shock†
100 J : 200 J : 360 J
or equivalent biphasic energy

If necessary, amiodarone 150 mg IV over 10 min, then 300 mg over 1 h and repeat shock

Doses throughout are based on an adult of average body weight
A starting dose of 6 mg adenosine is currently outside the UK licence for this agent.

* Note 1: Theophylline and related compounds block the effect of adenosine. Patients on dipyridamole, carbarnazepine, or with denervated hearts have a markedly exaggerated effect which may be hazardous

† Note 2: DC shock is always given under sedation/general anaesthesia.

** Note 3: Not to be used in patients receiving beta-blockers.

Atrial fibrillation algorithm

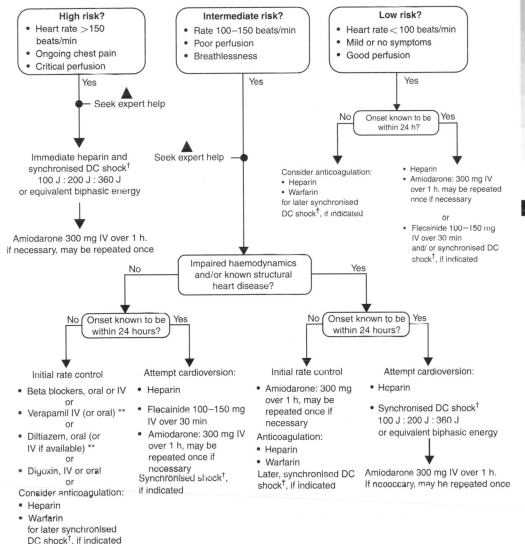

If appropriate, give oxygen and establish IV access

| **High risk?** |
| • Heart rate >150 beats/min |
| • Ongoing chest pain |
| • Critical perfusion |

Yes

— Seek expert help

Immediate heparin and synchronised DC shock†
100 J : 200 J : 360 J
or equivalent biphasic energy

Amiodarone 300 mg IV over 1 h. if necessary, may be repeated once

| **Intermediate risk?** |
| • Rate 100–150 beats/min |
| • Poor perfusion |
| • Breathlessness |

Yes

Seek expert help

Impaired haemodynamics and/or known structural heart disease?

No

Onset known to be within 24 hours?

No   Yes

Initial rate control
• Beta blockers, oral or IV
  or
• Verapamil IV (or oral) **
  or
• Diltiazem, oral (or IV if available) **
  or
• Digoxin, IV or oral
  or
Consider anticoagulation:
• Heparin
• Warfarin
for later synchronised DC shock†, if indicated

Attempt cardioversion:
• Heparin
• Flecainide 100–150 mg IV over 30 min
• Amiodarone: 300 mg IV over 1 h, may be repeated once if necessary
Synchronised shock†, if indicated

Yes

Onset known to be within 24 hours?

No   Yes

Initial rate control
• Amiodarone: 300 mg over 1 h, may be repeated once if necessary
Anticoagulation:
• Heparin
• Warfarin
Later, synchronised DC shock†, if indicated

Attempt cardioversion:
• Heparin
• Synchronised DC shock†
100 J : 200 J : 360 J
or equivalent biphasic energy

Amiodarone 300 mg IV over 1 h. If necessary, may be repeated once

| **Low risk?** |
| • Heart rate < 100 beats/min |
| • Mild or no symptoms |
| • Good perfusion |

Yes

No   Onset known to be within 24 h?   Yes

Consider anticoagulation:
• Heparin
• Warfarin
for later synchronised DC shock†, if indicated

• Heparin
• Amiodarone: 300 mg IV over 1 h. may be repeated once if necessary

or

• Flecainide 100–150 mg IV over 30 min
and/ or synchronised DC shock†, if indicated

Doses throughout are based on an adult of average body weight

† Note 1: DC shock is always given under sedation/general anaesthesia.
** Note 2: Not to be used in patients receiving beta-blockers.

Paediatric basic life support

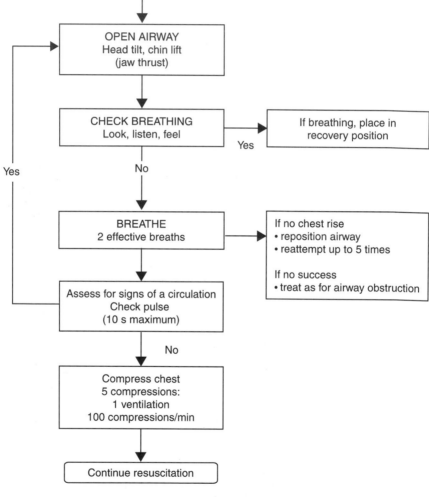

Paediatric advanced life support

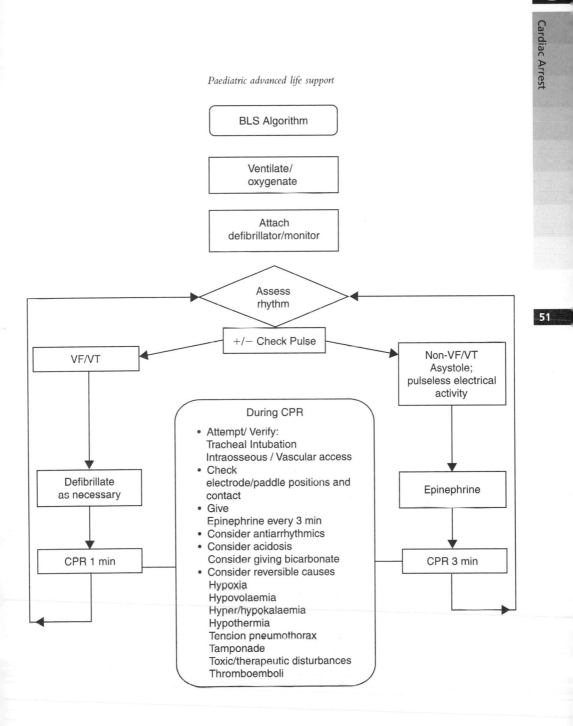

```
        ┌─────────────────────┐
        │   BLS Algorithm     │
        └─────────────────────┘
                  │
        ┌─────────────────────┐
        │    Ventilate/       │
        │    oxygenate        │
        └─────────────────────┘
                  │
        ┌─────────────────────┐
        │     Attach          │
        │ defibrillator/monitor│
        └─────────────────────┘
                  │
            ◇ Assess rhythm ◇
                  │
          +/- Check Pulse
```

VF/VT

Non-VF/VT
Asystole;
pulseless electrical
activity

Defibrillate
as necessary

Epinephrine

CPR 1 min

CPR 3 min

During CPR

- Attempt/ Verify:
  Tracheal Intubation
  Intraosseous / Vascular access
- Check
  electrode/paddle positions and
  contact
- Give
  Epinephrine every 3 min
- Consider antiarrhythmics
- Consider acidosis
  Consider giving bicarbonate
- Consider reversible causes
  Hypoxia
  Hypovolaemia
  Hyper/hypokalaemia
  Hypothermia
  Tension pneumothorax
  Tamponade
  Toxic/therapeutic disturbances
  Thromboemboli

Newborn life support

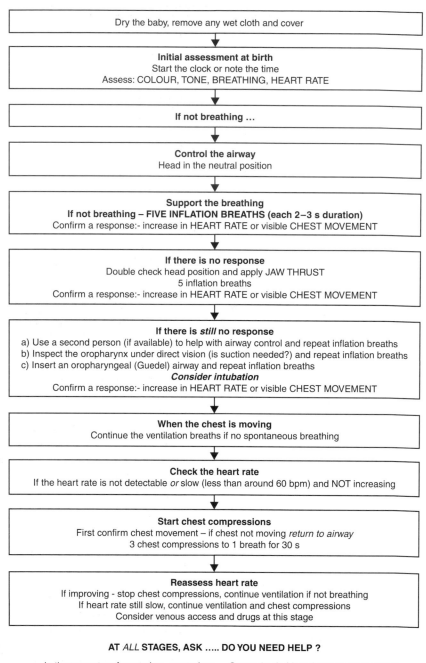

Dry the baby, remove any wet cloth and cover

Initial assessment at birth
Start the clock or note the time
Assess: COLOUR, TONE, BREATHING, HEART RATE

If not breathing ...

Control the airway
Head in the neutral position

Support the breathing
If not breathing – FIVE INFLATION BREATHS (each 2–3 s duration)
Confirm a response:- increase in HEART RATE or visible CHEST MOVEMENT

If there is no response
Double check head position and apply JAW THRUST
5 inflation breaths
Confirm a response:- increase in HEART RATE or visible CHEST MOVEMENT

If there is *still* no response
a) Use a second person (if available) to help with airway control and repeat inflation breaths
b) Inspect the oropharynx under direct vision (is suction needed?) and repeat inflation breaths
c) Insert an oropharyngeal (Guedel) airway and repeat inflation breaths
Consider intubation
Confirm a response:- increase in HEART RATE or visible CHEST MOVEMENT

When the chest is moving
Continue the ventilation breaths if no spontaneous breathing

Check the heart rate
If the heart rate is not detectable *or* slow (less than around 60 bpm) and NOT increasing

Start chest compressions
First confirm chest movement – if chest not moving *return to airway*
3 chest compressions to 1 breath for 30 s

Reassess heart rate
If improving - stop chest compressions, continue ventilation if not breathing
If heart rate still slow, continue ventilation and chest compressions
Consider venous access and drugs at this stage

AT *ALL* STAGES, ASK ..... DO YOU NEED HELP ?

In the presence of meconium, remember: Screaming babies:- have an open airway
                                            Floppy babies:-   have a look

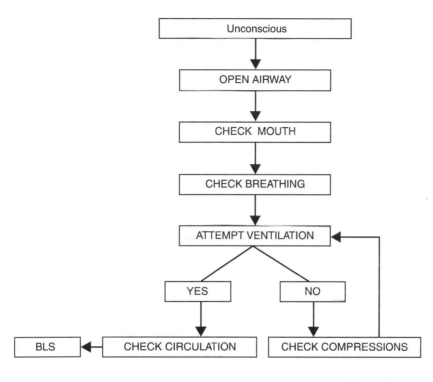

Management of choking in adults

```
                    Unconscious
                         │
                         ▼
                   OPEN AIRWAY
                         │
                         ▼
                  CHECK  MOUTH
                         │
                         ▼
                 CHECK BREATHING
                         │
                         ▼
              ATTEMPT VENTILATION  ◄────┐
                   │        │           │
                   ▼        ▼           │
                 YES       NO           │
                  │         │           │
                  ▼         ▼           │
   BLS ◄── CHECK CIRCULATION   CHECK COMPRESSIONS
```

During anaesthesia
Call for help, look for a cause
100% oxygen
Chest compressions 100/min
IPPV
Atropine 3 mg, epinephrine 500 g
Defibrillation

Cardiac arrest during anaesthesia. The peripheral pulse will normally not be palpable below 50 mmHg.

- Stop all anaesthetic agents. Check all causes of hypoxia and administer 100% oxygen. Check for hypovolaemia – give fluids and think of embolism. Note time.

- Alert resuscitation team and get defibrillator.

- Commence external chest compression (ECC) over lower sternum – 100 compressions/min. Fifty per cent of the cycle must be compression. Epinephrine 1 mg IV or more through tracheal tube. Atropine 3 mg if vagal tone high; seen with high spinal blocks and certain surgical stimuli.

- Ventilate via tracheal tube (TT). Check oxygen supply, machine, ventilator, breathing system and tracheal are sound. If in doubt replace TT. If intubation was difficult use a bougie or catheter through the tube before removing tube and check it stops at the carina at 35–40 cm, if it passes 60 cm it is in the oesophagus. Ventilate manually with a simple breathing system e.g. Ambu bag and one-way valve, or mouth to tube, provide oxygen from a cylinder. Use a different anaesthetic machine. Single person chest compression 15:2 chest inflations, 2 people 5:1. Using 100 compressions/min.

- Monitor ECG. If ECG not available, treat as for VF. If VF defibrillate. Place one electrode to right of the sternum, below clavicle, and the other on the anterior axillary line over the fifth left intercostal space. Commence DC shock at 200 J. Repeat once and then increase to 360 J. Maintain CPR between shocks. Large bore cannula IV access or central vein if hypovolaemic. Many essential drugs may be given down the TT. If VF still persists give lidocaine 100 mg IV or 200 mg via TT and repeat DC shock (360 J). If VF is low amplitude (fine) give 1 mg epinephrine (10 ml of 1/10,000) IV or 2 mg (20 ml of 1/10,000) via TT, and repeat DC shock (360 J). If arrest has lasted for 15 min consider stopping resuscitation unless hypothermic. Take arterial blood sample for blood gas acid–base analysis and K^+ estimation. If VF still present, consider further lidocaine and antiarrhythmic. Then repeat DC shock (360 J). If defibrillation is successful, a lidocaine infusion may be necessary to maintain a stable rhythm.

- ECG asystole. Many essential drugs may be given IV or through TT in the following sequence and doses: epinephrine 1 mg(10 ml of 1:10,000) IV or 2 mg (20 ml of 1:10,000) TT. Atropine 1 mg IV or 2 mg TT. Isoprenaline infusion 0.5–10 g/min IV or 4–8 g/min TT. Calcium chloride 10 ml 10% IV. If serum potassium known to be raised, give calcium initially. Calcium is of doubtful value if arrest due to primary cardiac cause. Repeat doses of all these drugs may be necessary. If ineffective, consider pacing.

- When blood chemistry results available: correct serum potassium as follows: <3 mmol/l give 20 mmol KCl, slowly; >5 mmol/l give 10 ml 10% calcium chloride.

- Repeat blood gas, acid–base and potassium determination every 30 min.

- If resuscitation is successful admit patient to ICU or CCU. Dopamine, dobutamine or norepinephrine infusion if evidence of low cardiac output. X-ray chest – look for fractured ribs and pneumothorax. Measure urine output and consider mannitol 0.5 g/kg over 10–20 min. Check Hb, WBC, electrolytes and acid–base state.

Infusion regimens, best by IV pump.

- Lidocaine 500 mg in 500 ml fluid = 1 mg/ml.

- Isoprenaline 2 mg in 500 ml fluid = 4 μg/ml.

- Standard drip sets (e.g. Avon, Baxter) = 15 drops/ml.

- Microdrip sets (e.g. Soluset) = 60 drops/ml.

Carotid sinus massage

- Patients with AV and SA node disease and who may be sensitive to parasympathetic stimulation are prone to bradycardia and may benefit from preoperative pacing.

- Stimulating the carotid sinus preoperatively can confirm the presence of severe SA node disease when there are minimum ECG changes.

- Used to terminate paroxysmal SVT, relieve the pain of angina pectoris and reduce LVF.

- The development of AV block or ectopic beats may indicate digoxin toxicity.[18]

Prone resuscitation

- When a patient collapses in the prone position, during surgery, reversed precordial compression can be used when it would take time to turn the patient supine.

- Reversed precordial compression is performed with one hand placed on the patient's back over the mid-thoracic spine and is used to compress the thorax rhythmically.

- The other hand, clenched in a fist, is held over the lower third of the sternum to stabilise the chest.

- The hands should be changed over frequently as they become tired.[19,20]

Cervical collar

- Two patients had a rise in intracranial pressure following the application of a rigid neck collar. Neck stabilisation is essential following an accident but if a patient deteriorates it is possible that the collar is impeding venous drainage and it should be replaced by sand bags and other means of fixation.[21]

Chest Drains

A non-return valve can be made from a condom, with a slit end, over the tube or more usually an underwater seal.

- Chest drain can be connected in a variety of ways to the underwater seal bottles which should be 1 m below the level of the patient. The intrathoracic pressure must reach 100 cmH$_2$O negative to suck water from the bottle into the tube before it reaches the chest. At this point the column of water would be exerting a negative pressure of 100 cmH$_2$O on the intrapleural space to expand the lung.

- A single bottle should have the drain tube from the patient 2–5 cm below the water surface. Any increase in depth of water or accumulation of fluid in the drain will raise

intrapleural pressure, which further limits fluid drainage and expansion of the lung. The bottle should be emptied of drained fluid at regular intervals. The volume of water between the surface and the depth of the tube should be sufficient to fill the pleural drain during a maximum inspiration. A second tube acts as a vent (Figure 14).

- A two-bottle system allows blood or fluid to collect in the first bottle while the level of water in the second bottle remains constant. The first bottle increases the total dead space air which is compressible. Moving with the pleural air it will slow the re-expansion of the lung (Figure 15).

- A three-bottle system can be used for suction. The depth of the central control tube regulates the maximum negative pressure that can be applied (Figure 16).

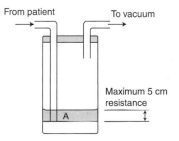

Figure 14 – Single bottle underwater seal (Vol. A = total volume to fill 1 m drain tube).

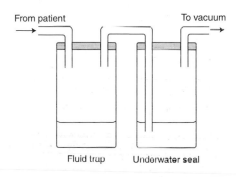

Figure 15 – Two-bottles fluid trap and underwater seal.

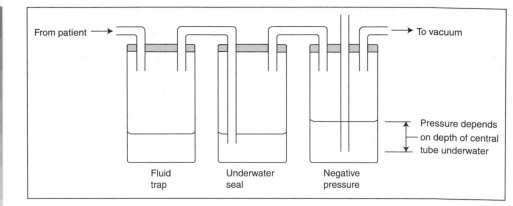

Figure 16 – Third bottle used to determine negative intrathoracic pressure.

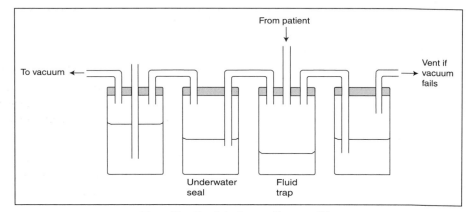

Figure 17 – Fourth bottle vents if vacuum fails.

- Adding a fourth safety bottle will vent the system and relieve any pressure build-up should the suction fail[22] (Figure 17).

Chest X-rays

The presentation of the X-ray is important before any diagnosis can be made.

- *Penetration.* The upper 4–6 thoracic vertebrae should be visible through the mediastinal shadow. If more are seen the film is overpenetrated, if fewer or no vertebral bodies are seen the film is underpenetrated. Underpenetration may lead to a lung field appearing whiter than it is, overpenetration may give the appearance of hyperinflation.

- *Centred.* The distances between the clavicular heads and the spine of the vertebra should be equal on both sides. Check that the spine is not kyphoscoliotic. If the spine is curved and parallax is seen (more than one of every edge), it is likely that the patient will have unequal lung volumes.

- A film should be taken in deep inspiration which will flatten the diaphragms and show at least six anterior ribs and eight posterior ribs.

- *PA*. An elective chest X-ray is taken with the patient standing, shoulders abducted and the anterior chest wall against the film. This film will show the scapulae out of the lung field. The X-rays are transmitted from the posterior chest wall. Anterior chest structures, such as the heart are not magnified. The heart diameter should be less than half of the chest diameter, with exceptions (below). An AP film will tend to magnify anterior chest structures.

- The X-ray should be viewed against a white light which lights the whole film. It is useful to turn the film through 90° to make the lung edge of a pneumothorax more obvious and through 180° (upside down) to bring fractured ribs into prominence.

Systematic examination of the film

- *Trachea*. Should be central. Deviations may be due to a neck lesion, thyroid gland, apical fibrosis or kyphoscoliosis. There should be air in the trachea. Narrowing or deviation may suggest a difficult intubation. Ask for a CT scan.

- *Diaphragm*. The right diaphragm dome is normally higher than the left due to the position of the liver. The relative position of the domes of the diaphragms should be considered with other findings to make a rational diagnosis. Lung collapse will lead to elevation of the diaphragm on the affected side but lung hyperinflation on the other side, which depresses that dome. Symmetrical hyperinflation leads to flattening of both diaphragms. Elevation of a diaphragm may be due to a subdiaphragmatic lesion. In the presence of trauma the right diaphragm rises due to a liver haematoma and the left rises with splenic disease.

- Hilar area for opacities.

- Vascular markings increased in oedema.

- Lung fields for symmetry of air entry, lesions, bullae.

- Bones of the arm, ribs and clavicles for fractures, secondary deposits, notching of coarctation; osteomalacia, inadequate mineralisation of the osteoid framework in pelvis, ribs, long bones (looser's zone = linear areas of lower density associated with osteomalacia); osteoporosis, thin bone, reduced bone mass and fractures.

- Soft tissue for surgical emphysema.

Abnormal chest X-rays

Emphysema

- Hyperinflated lungs, over eight posterior ribs and over six anterior ribs visible, ribs flattened and the spaces between widened, diaphragms flattened, large lucent areas (bullae).

- The diagnosis of chronic obstructive airways disease (COAD) is made when there is evidence of bronchospasm and emphysema.

Collapse and consolidation

On affected side:

- Trachea deviated towards affected side.

- Mediastinal shift towards affected side. Diaphragm elevated.

- Space between ribs narrowed (crowding).

On opposite side:

- Compensatory emphysema. Ribs splayed. Diaphragm depressed.

Causes: infection including tuberculosis, tumours, tracheo-bronchial lymph nodes and aspiration. The causes refer to both On affected and On opposite side.

Blockage

Right middle lobe bronchus

- Loss of right atrial outline or triangular shadow at right hilum.

Right lower lobe bronchus

- No loss of right atrial outline.

Causes: secretions, foreign bodies in bronchus e.g. peanuts in children.

Pleural effusion

- Need >300 ml to be obvious. Over 500 ml will show as blunting of the costo-phrenic angle on an erect film.

- A film taken with the patient supine may show nothing, or an increased whiteness due to lack of penetration of the affected lung as the fluid is spread over the surface of the pleura.

- Large effusion – opaque hemithorax. Mediastinum shifted away as the fluid increases.

Fibrosis

- *Local*: streaky shadowing. Reduced lung volume. Mediastinal shift towards affected side.

- *General*: honeycomb. Diffuse shadows with multiple translucencies a few mm in diameter.

Round shadows

- Carcinoma, primary or secondary. Tuberculoma. Lung abscess or hydatid cyst with or without a fluid level.

- Encapsulated interlobar effusion (usually horizontal fissure). Arterial–venous malformation adjacent to a vascular shadow, aspergilosis, rheumatoid nodules.

- Rare: bronchial carcinoid, cylindroma, chondroma, lipoma.

Miliary mottling

Multiple opacities 1–3 mm in size.

- Many causes e.g. miliary TB, pneumoconiosis, sarcoidosis, fibrosing alveolitis, pulmonary oedema – usually perihilar with large fluffy shadows.

- Rare: pulmonary microlithiasis.

Oesophagus

Findings: dilated oesophagus, fluid level in neck, no fundal stomach gas shadow.

Due to achalasia – no peristalsis in oesophagus with failure in relaxation of smooth muscle. Oesophageal diverticulae occur at three levels: above the upper oesophageal sphincter (oesophageal pouch); near middle oesophagus; above lower oesophageal sphincter.

Findings: hydropneumothorax.

Due to Mallory–Weiss tear at oesophago-gastric junction. Oesophageal rupture associated with violent vomiting and often alcohol ingestion.

Mediastinal shadow

No air seen between the mediastinum and the lesion.

- Causes: Hodgkin lymphoma or non-Hodgkin lymphoma. Clarify lung involvement with a CT scan.

- Multiple myeloma. Clarify by presence of lytic lesions in skull and other bones.

- Sarcoidosis.

- Carcinoma of prostate, thyroid, breast. Bone involvement with lung, breast, prostate and less often kidney and thyroid.

- Need a lateral film or other examination for lesions of the pericardium, oesophagus or spinal cord.

Bronchiectasis

An X-ray diagnosis shows dilatation of the main bronchi with consolidation, a honeycomb pattern and bronchial wall thickening.

Heart

Trace the outline and note the shape, size and position. Cardiac shadow maximum diameter divided by total thoracic diameter (CT) should be <50% or up to 15.5 cm. Increase in cardiac shadow usually due to dilation of one or both ventricles, but may be a normal finding in neonates, kyphoscoliosis, funnel chest and athletes.

Normal outline

From top left, clockwise: aorta, left atrial appendage, left ventricle, right ventricle border on diaphragm, right atrium makes the border of the right mediastinum with the superior vena cava above.

Abnormalities

- Pericardial effusion: globular shadow, sharp edges, no vascular markings.

- Heart failure: large heart and increased vascular changes.

- Left atrial enlargement (mitral stenosis): straight edge to left border between aorta and left ventricle (left border may also appear straight with left lower lobe collapse). Right heart border projects into right lower lung field. Double atrial shadow to right of sternum.

- Splayed carina due to elevation of left main bronchus. Lateral X-ray shows enlarged left atrium bulging backwards, displacing the left main stem bronchus.

- Left ventricle enlargement: CT diameter increased and increased convexity of left border. Causes: left ventricular enlargement, ventricular aneurysm.

- Right ventricle enlargement (congenital heart) CT increased. Apex upward displacement. Lateral view; enlargement anteriorly for right ventricle, posteriorly for left ventricle.

Aortic dilatation – prominent aortic shadow. To right of mediastinum between right atrium and superior vena cava.

Enlarged pulmonary artery = pulmonary hypertension and pulmonary artery stenosis with left to right shunt. Seen as a bulge on the left-hand border of the mediastinum below the aortic knuckle.

Calcification

- Pericardial calcification plaque. Opacity in A/V groove.

- Vascular calcification: common in aorta over 40 years of age. Coronary artery calcification proximal left coronary artery.

- Long-standing rheumatic heart disease or bicuspid aortic valve disease. Usually in mitral or aortic valves. Lateral film. Line joining carina to sterno-phrenic angle – aortic valve calcification on this line. Mitral valve below and behind this line.

- Myocardial calcification with infarction.

Pulmonary vascular markings (NB markings are vascular not bronchovascular).

1. Pulmonary plethora with a left to right shunt. Increased size of right lower lobe artery (normal 16 mm diameter).

2. Pulmonary oligaemia – reduced vascular markings in: pulmonary embolism, pulmonary stenosis, Fallot's tetralogy.

3. Pulmonary hypertension changes symmetrical – enlarged right heart, prominent pulmonary arteries, late sign pruning of peripheral vessels – Eisenmenger syndrome. Primary cause rare. Secondary to congenital heart disease.

4. Pulmonary venous hypertension.

   • Normal pressure 5–14 mmHg.

   • Mild 15–20 mmHg. Isolated dilated vessels in upper zone.

   • Pressure 21–30 mmHg. Interstitial oedema seen as fluid in interlobular fissures, interlobular septa (Kerley B lines), pleural spaces. Indistinct hilar region and haziness of lung fields.

   • Pressure over 30 mmHg. Alveolar oedema – consolidated mottling of lung fields, pleural effusion.

Role of Doppler echocardiography to assess:

• Ventricular wall function.

• Ejection fraction normally >55–70% depending on operator. That is ventricular volume 100 ml, stroke volume 70 ml. Poor if <40%, or large ventricle.

• Right ventricular pressure and severity of pulmonary hypertension.

• Nature of congenital heart disease and left-sided cardiac conditions.

• Severity of valve stenosis or reflux.

• Dissection of the aorta ideally with transoesophageal echocardiography.

• Pericardial effusion and guide aspiration.

Features of specific conditions

• Inhaled foreign body. Collapsed or hyperinflated lung. Opaque lung markings if collapsed lung. Hyperlucent with depressed diaphragm if ball valve effect and air trapping on expiration.

• COAD. CXR shows hyperinflated emphysema, possibly bullae. Vitalograph shows obstructive pattern.

• Thrombo-embolism reduced vascular markings.

Children and Anaesthesia

Children with acute infection should have elective surgery postponed. A chronic runny nose or cough will make the airway irritable and an anticholinergic should be used.

Age	BP	Pulse rate/min	Respiratory rate/min
Birth	80/45	140 (90–200)	40
1 year	95/65	120 (75–150)	20–30
7 years	105/65	100 (70–135)	20
Puberty	120/70	85 (55–120)	10–14

Tracheal tubes

Age	Tube ID (mm)	Nasal tube length (cm)
Premature	3–2.5	
Term	3.5	11.8
6 months	4	12.6
6–24 months	4.5	13.6–15.2

Tube length relates better to age than weight. Listen for a small leak with a stethoscope over the larynx. If a child needs re-intubation choose a smaller diameter tube after the first time. Laryngeal damage is associated with the number of intubations not the duration of intubation.

Respiratory distress in child

Look at colour, heart rate, respiratory rate, conscious level. Differentiate inspiratory stridor due to Croup and Epiglottitis.

Congenital stridor is relieved by holding the chin forward or nursing prone.

	Croup	Epiglottitis
Cause	Parainfluenza virus	Haemophilus influenza Type B
Age	Under 3 years	Under 5 years
Progress	Days	Hours
Debility	Mild	Febrile, ill
Sedation	Given	Not until intubated
Steroids	May reduce oedema	Not indicated
Antibiotics	No	Yes
Intubation	Rare	Always intubate early if in doubt

Asthma – expiratory wheeze. As in adult, intubate if in doubt especially if exhausted and unable to talk or cough. Do not send to another department.

Haemoglobin

At birth 20 g/dl HbF. Three months 10 g/dl and may not rise further until puberty due to diet and growth.

Blood volume. At birth 100 ml/kg, childhood 80 ml/kg, puberty 70 ml/kg.

Cyanosis during Anaesthesia

Check
- Anaesthetic machine and breathing system
- Airway
- Patient

Cyanosis. Over 5 g Hb desaturated/100 ml of blood. Is the patient breathing spontaneously or paralysed?

1. *Breathing spontaneous or paralysed and ventilated*

Chest not moving – connect mask or tracheal tube to self-inflating bag and 100% oxygen or blow down TT via filter. Exclude oesophageal intubation.

Chest easy to inflate with self-inflating bag:

A. Fault in ventilator, gas supply or breathing system. Exclude by continuing with self-inflating bag and cylinder oxygen.

Chest impossible or difficult to inflate:

B. Fault in airway or tracheal tube

- Outside larynx e.g. oesophagus.

- Blocked, kinked – inspect with laryngoscope and pass stout catheter with oxygen attached through tube to check patency. It will pass more than 40 cm if the tube is in the oesophagus.

- Herniated cuff – check pharynx dry, then deflate cuff.

- In a bronchus – withdraw TT tube. Feel cuff in neck.

C. Fault in patient

RS

Exclude: one-lung anaesthesia, bronchospasm, pulmonary oedema, pneumothorax, haemothorax, aspiration, laryngospasm, hyperpyrexia.

- One-lung anaesthsia – listen to chest.
- Bronchospasm – listen for expiratory wheeze.
- Fluid in alveoli – listen for crepitations or wheeze, look for blood stained tracheal fluid.
- Pneumothorax – absent breath sounds over affected side. Usually one sided. Check for tracheal deviation indicating tension.
- Haemothorax – absent breath sounds over dependent part of lung.
- Aspiration – history of vomiting.
- Laryngospasm – inspiratory wheeze. Try midazolam IV, LA throat spray, re-intubate.

- Hyperpyrexia – check temperature, expired oxygen and carbon dioxide.

CVS

Ensure adequate cardiac output. Check pulse. Exclude anaphylactic reaction, fluid depletion, arrhythmia, embolism.

2. *Breathing spontaneously*

Chest not moving

- Treat as for paralysed patient.
- Attach to self-inflating bag.

Chest moving

- Eliminate machine causes by using 100% oxygen from a cylinder.
- Airway check pharynx, insert airway, intubate.
- If intubated check oesophagus and capnograph for expired carbon dioxide.
- Pass bougie through tracheal tube, if it passed more than 40 cm it is in the oesophagus.
- Inadequate ventilation due to low minute ventilation, low oxygen tension, excess of drugs, one lung ventilation, often oxygen saturation around 85%.
- Check pulse and BP for low cardiac output.

3. *Paralysed and ventilated patient*

Chest not moving

- Isolate the patient from the anaesthetic machine by using a self-inflating bag with cylinder oxygen.
- 100% oxygen from cylinder if malignant hyperthermia or defective gas supply.
- Airway. Intubate. If intubated check oesophagus and expired carbon dioxide.

If bougie or catheter in tracheal tube (TT) passes more than 40 cm tube is in the oesophagus.

Circulatory causes of cyanosis

- fluid loss,
- reduced venous return,
- pump failure,
- obstruction to vena cava or aorta,
- massive embolism,
- severe hypersensitivity reaction.

Fault in oxygen supply to the patient

- Source of oxygen exhausted.
- Oxygen diluted with other gas e.g. carbon dioxide.
- Machine leaking O_2, measure FiO_2 with oxygen meter.
- Pipeline – cross connection – check with oxygen analyser.
- Breathing system
  - Fresh gas supply inadequate.
  - Leak.
  - Incorrectly assembled.

Miscellaneous causes

- Malignant hyperpyrexia, check low expired oxygen, high expired carbon dioxide.
- Methaemoglobinaemia. Give methylene blue 1 mg/kg IV. Patient will remain blue but oxygenation will improve.

If the cause of cyanosis is not obvious
- Use self inflating bag with cylinder oxygen
- Or use attendant's expired air
- Change anaesthetic machine
- Change tracheal tube

References

1. Asai T. Fixation of capnograph sampling tube to a Hudson mask. *Anaesthesia* 1994; **49:** 745.

2. Skjellerup N. Respiratory monitoring for regional anaesthesia. *Anaesthesia* 1994; **49:** 1097.

3. Reah G. Nasal cannulae and capnography for all. *Anaesthesia* 1995; **50:** 95.

4. Goldman JM. A simple easy, and inexpensive method for monitoring $ETCO_2$ through nasal cannulae. *Anesthesiology* 1987; **67:** 606.

5. Reid MF, Matthews A. A simple arrangement to sample expired gas in small children. *Anaesthesia* 1988; **43:** 902–3.

6. Ooi TK. A new use for the hole in the bag. *Anaesthesia* 1989; **44:** 79.

7. Ball AJ. Paediatric capnography. *Anaesthesia* 1995; **50:** 833–4.

8. Masher SJ. Capnography in babies and small children. *Anaesthesia* 1994; **49:** 1096–7.

9. Petrioanu G, Widjaja B, Bergler WF. Detection of oesophageal intubation: can the "cola complication" be potentially lethal? *Anaesthesia* 1992; **47:** 70–1.

10. Zbinden S, Schupfer G. Detection of oesophageal intubation: the cola complication. *Anaesthesia* 1989; **44:** 81.

11. Schuller L, Bovill JG, Nijveld A. End-tidal carbon dioxide concentrations as an indicator of pulmonary blood flow during closed heart surgery in children. *British Journal of Anaesthesia* 1985; **57:** 1257–9.

12. Nichols KP, Benumof JL. Biphasic carbon dioxide excretion waveform from a patient with severe kyphoscoliosis. *Anesthesiology* 1989; **71:** 986–7.

13. Fazlollah TM, Tosone SR. End-tidal carbon dioxide monitoring may help diagnosis of H-type tracheal-oesophageal fistula. *Anesthesiology* 1995; **83:** 878.

14. Gozal Y, Robinson ST. An unusual capnogram. *Anesthesiology* 1997; **87:** 453.

15. Martin M, Zupan J. Unusual end-tidal CO_2 waveform. *Anesthesiology* 1987; **66:** 712–13.

16. Hilberman M. Capnometer readings at high altitude. *Anesthesiology* 1990; **73:** 354–5.

17. Baskett PJF, Strunin L. Resuscitation, postgraduate education issue. *British Journal of Anaesthesia* 1997; 79.

18. McConachie I. Value of pre-operative carotid sinus massage. *Anaesthesia* 1987; **42:** 636–8.

19. Sun WZ, Huang FY, Kung KL, Fan SZ, Chen TL. Successful cardiopulmonary resuscitation of two patients in the prone position using reversed precordial compression. *Anesthesiology* 1992; **77:** 202–4.

20. Dequin PF et al. Cardiopulmonary resuscitation in the prone position: Kouwenhoven revisited. *Intensive Care Medicine* 1996; **22:** 1272.

21. Craig GR, Nielson MS. Rigid cervical collars and intracranial pressure. *Intensive Care Medicine* 1991; **17:** 504–5.

22. Kam AC, O'Brien M, Kam PCA. Pleural drainage systems. *Anaesthesia* 1993; **48:** 154–61.

Diabetes

Check for arterial disease, sympathetic and peripheral neuropathy, renal function, cataract and glycosylated haemoglobin for chronicity of hyperglycaemia.

There are a number of regimes for managing diabetic patients. Alberti[1] suggested a regime of glucose 10 g with 2 units insulin and KCl 2 mmol every hour. This is modified, depending on the initial blood glucose. If the blood glucose is under 6 mmol/l: 5 units insulin is added to 500 ml dextrose (10%) with KCl 10 mmol over 6 h. If blood glucose is over 6 mmol/l then 10 units insulin is added, if blood glucose is over 15 mmol/l then 15 units insulin is added to 500 ml glucose (10%).

Management of non-insulin dependent diabetic for surgery[2,3]

- Stop oral hypoglycaemics the night before surgery, chlorpropamide earlier.

- Assess CVS and ECG.

- Morning of surgery. First case on list.

- Start infusion of 5% dextrose 1000 ml over 8 h to prevent hypoglycaemia. Add 27 mmol/l potassium.

- Check BM stix every 3 h but hourly during anaesthesia and other periods of unconsciousness. Monitor serum potassium.

- Give insulin e.g. Purin neutral subcutaneously.

BM stix every 3 h	Insulin
0–6.5	Nil
6.6–9.0	5 units
9.1–11.0	6 units
11.1–17.0	8 units
If above 17.0	10 units

For minor/day surgery, blood glucose of 5–12 mmol/l is acceptable.[4] An insulin and glucose with potassium regime (GIK) has a predictable effect. If the surgery is atraumatic, short and the diabetes is well controlled a GIK regime may be replaced by a regime such as:

- Continue with oral hypoglycaemics on the night before surgery.

- Give light breakfast no less than 2 h preoperatively.

- First case on list in morning, no IV regime.

- Monitor blood glucose every 3 h until returns to drinking.

- Any complications switch to insulin, glucose, and potassium regime.

Insulin dependent diabetic for surgery

- Omit morning dose of regular insulin.

- Ten per cent dextrose 1000 ml every 8 h or 100 ml/h through dedicated line, with 20–27 mmol potassium.

- Sliding scale insulin (subcutaneously). Measure BM stix hourly during unconsciousness and 3 hourly when awake.

BM stix	Purin neutral insulin
0–4.5	0 units
4.6–6.5	2 units
6.6–9	4 units
9.1–11	6 units
11.1–17	8 units
17–28	10 units
Over 28	Seek expert advice

The alternative to subcutaneous insulin is an infusion regime.

- Thousand ml saline (0.9%) with 80 mmol potassium over 24 h via a dedicated cannula. Dextrose 5–10% 1 l every 8 h or 500 ml every 6 h.

- Insulin infusions. The normal requirement for insulin IV is 1–2 units/h. This can be given by continuous infusion using a syringe pump, or adding to a dextrose 5% or 10%

infusion. Boluses of insulin IV are destroyed by liver insulinase within minutes.

Diabetic ketoacidosis

Monitor every 2 h blood glucose, sodium and potassium. When blood glucose <12 mmol/l monitor every 4 h. Bladder catheter, if no urine (Table 3).

If patient has sodium >155 meq/l and normal pH they have a hyperosmolar non-ketotic state. Give half-normal saline, half the insulin dose and subcutaneous heparin 5000 units.

Drugs

Aerosol drug applications

Uses: Bronchodilation, resuscitation, analgesia, sedation and for ENT surgery. Patient who is nervous, mentally disturbed, frightened of needles and anaesthetics. Poor venous access.

- Drugs that have been given as aerosols include: local anaesthetics, cocaine, midazolam for premedication, epinephrine (adrenaline), salbutamol, atropine, hyoscine; ketamine and fentanyl for pain relief.

- Advantages: rapid onset, alternative to IV for resuscitation – adrenaline (epinephrine) and atropine. Self-administration, no first pass effect, ideal for beta 2 agonist bronchodilators with less cardiac effect than IV.

- Problems: variable patient compliance leading to variable dosing, bitter taste of many drugs, correct size of particles.

Methods

- Aerosol fits mouth piece or mask.

- Aerosol fitted into a syringe and the piston used to activate the aerosol.

- Bolus of drug injected into proximal tracheal tube.

- An intravenous cannula fitted to an aerosol or syringe and pass into the distal tracheal tube.

Table 3 – Management of diabetic ketoacidosis

Infusion	Blood glucose >12 mmol/l	Insulin	Bicarbonate
Normal saline 1 l, 1 h 1 l, 2 h 1 l, 4 h	Potassium <3.5 add 40 mmol/l 3.5–5 add 27 mmol/l	Humulin S, Human Actrapid, Human Velosulin 20 units IM then 5 units every 1 h Increase to 10 units after 2 h if no change in blood glucose. or 6 units/h continuous infusion IV if no change in blood glucose after 2 h 10 units/h	(H^+) <100 nil (H^+) >100 give 50 mmol $NaHCO_3$ over 30 min Check pH 30 min later Repeat up to 3 times Give extra potassium 10 mmol KCl for each 50 mmol $NaHCO_3$
When blood glucose <12 mmol/l 5% glucose 1 l/8 h	Potassium as above	Short acting insulin Insulin IV infusion 1–3 units/h IM 5 units (2–10) every 3 h	

- Aerosol or a syringe pushed through a rubber sleeve fitted over a gas sampling port in an airway connection.

Drug dosage

Dose for children

- It is often recommended that drug dosage in children should be calculated with reference to body weight. There is no direct correlation between weight and drug dosage.

- A rule for clinical use is up to 30 kg, a child's drug dose (weight $\times$ 2)% of an adult dose; over 30 kg (weight $+$ 30)% of an adult dose.[5]

Drug infusion rates

- If the patient's weight is W kg, add 6 times W in milligrams of the drug to a burette or infusion device, make the volume up to 100 ml. Then the setting of the infusion device in ml/h will be numerically the same as the dose of the drug administered in μg/kg/min. If the device acts as a drip counter delivering 60 drops/ml, then using the same dilution drops/min is equivalent to μg/kg/min.[6]

- Calculations for a strength of solution can be made from $1000Y = 60XVW$, $X =$ dose rate (μg/ml/kg/min), $Y =$ the amount of drug (mg) within the total volume of solution, $V =$ total volume (ml) of solution, $W =$ weight (kg) of patient. The equation can be rearranged so that if the volume is to be fixed at say 50 ml over 60 min, the amount of drug to be added, Y mg $= 60XVW/1000$.[7]

Drug interactions leading to prolonged action

- Cytochrome P450 catalyses the N-demethylation of erythromycin. The erythromycin breath test measures the ability of the patient to perform this demethylation. In 30 patients there was a four- to six-fold range of breath test values, indicating marked individual variability. Cytochrome P450 IIIA appears to have a broad unimodal distribution of enzyme activity in the population. There is in vitro evidence that midazolam is also metabolised by cytochrome P450 IIIA. Interactions with a prolongation of duration of effect in some patients given erythromycin, midazolam, alfentanyl and theophylline may be accounted for by this individual variation in P450 IIIA activity.[8]

Osmolarity

- Solutions with an osmolarity of less than 130 mosmol/kg water cause haemolysis. The amount depends on the volume administered. Drugs with low osmolarities: Fentanyl 0.05 mg/ml 0 mosmol/kg, Morphine HCl 10 mg/ml 54 mosmol/kg, Propranolol 1 mg/ml 12 mosmol/kg, Ranitidine 10 mg/ml 59 mosmol/kg. The osmolarities of drug preparations varies depending on the manufacturer. Some toxic effects of drugs may be due to the volume of fluid and cell hypoxia rather than drug effect.[9]

Specific drugs and conditions

Diltiazem and ventricular fibrillation

- Diltiazem, a calcium channel blocker, suppresses ventricular fibrillation induced by myocardial ischaemia in animals. Diltiazem 5 mg IV relieved ventricular fibrillation after 5 episodes of defibrillation and lidocaine 50 mg in a 75-year-old man.[10]

Hiccups

Hiccup can be a problem during light anaesthesia and recovery.

Remedies include

- Drugs: Ketamine, methylphenidate, ephedrine, edrophonium, chlorpromazine, doxapram, anticonvulsants and muscle relaxants.

- Nasopharyngeal stimulation to inhibit vagal afferent impulses. This can be achieved by passing 5 ml of ice cold saline into the nasopharynx.

- Sedated patients rather than anaesthetised may breath ammonium chloride (smelling salts) broken under the nose.[11]

- Apply CPAP at 25–35 cmH$_2$O with the patient breathing spontaneously, induced by a flow of oxygen through a face mask. This terminated the hiccups in 16 patients within 15 s.[12]

LA for myringotomy

- Fifty-six Honduran children had topical EMLA cream applied to the tympanic membrane with cotton wool tipped swabs and a tympanocentesis was performed 30–40 min later. It is also suggested that prilocaine and lidocaine are not toxic to the auditory nerve.[13] This may be used for postoperative pain relief.

MAC of anaesthetics

MAC50 is the minimum alveolar concentration at which 50% of the subjects do not respond to a painful stimulus. MAC90 is a more useful measure of anaesthetic need, being the concentration at which 90% do not respond. MAC90 is MAC50 × 1.5.

- The MAC of an anaesthetic gas mixture is the sum of the MACs of the component parts. If 1.2% isoflurane is 1.0 MAC and 50% N$_2$O in O$_2$ is 0.5 MAC, then 0.6% isoflurane with 50% N$_2$O = 1.0 MAC.

The reason is that 0.6% isoflurane is 0.5 MAC and the N$_2$O is 0.5 MAC, added together they make 1.0 MAC. Thus 1.8% isoflurane in 50% N$_2$O will be 2.0 MAC.[14]

Anaesthetic	MAC	O/G PC	MAC × O/G PC
Isoflurane	1.2	90	108
Enflurane	1.8	96	178
Halothane	0.76	225	170
Desflurane	6.0	20	120
Sevoflurane	2.0	60	120

MAC varies by ±15% of the mean. If all volatile anaesthetic agents act at one, lipid soluble, site the multiple of MAC × oil/gas partition coefficient (O/G PC) would be constant. The multiple of MAC and O/G PC is not constant and therefore the theory that all volatile anaesthetics act at one hydrophobic site is not tenable.[15] The figures suggest two mechanisms of action.

Magnesium sulphate

Uses: pre-eclampsia and eclampsia, status asthmaticus, tetanus and SVT.

Doses of magnesium sulphate vary from a bolus of 2 or 3 g IV to 20 g in the first hour to facilitate IPPV in severe status asthmaticus. An infusion of up to 25 g infused over 24 h has been used.[16]

An increase in magnesium ions will cause muscle weakness, areflexia and potentiate non-depolarising muscle relaxants. Monitor reflexes, respiration and serum levels (see also page 117, Obstetrics – eclampsia).

Porphyria

A genetic deficiency in haem production resulting in the overproduction of porphyrin or a precursor.[17,18] The lack of haem aggravates the situation by inhibiting alpha-aminolaevulinic acid synthetase leading to an accumulation of porphobilinogen.

The disease causes constipation, vomiting and colic, depression and other psychological changes, photophobia, neuropathy bulbar and respiratory failure.

Any drug which induces enzymes will aggravate an attach. Avoid barbiturates, propofol,[19] phenothiazines, tricyclic antidepressants, MAOI and probably volatile agents. Also sulphonamides, anticonvulsants, alcohol and oral contraceptives. An anaesthetic can be given using midazolam, opioids, ketamine, NSAIDs, nitrous oxide and muscle relaxants with atropine and neostigmine; bupivacaine and procaine. The patient should avoid fasting and dehydration by giving IV glucose.

Premedication

- Young children accept an oral dose of ketamine 6 mg/kg mixed with a cola flavoured soft drink given 20–30 min before induction of anaesthesia. It provides satisfactory sedation without side effects. Most drugs, including ketamine are bitter if taken alone.[20]

- A lozenge of fentanyl citrate 15–20 μg/kg given 45 min preoperatively produces sedation and facilitates the induction of anaesthesia but decreases respiratory rate and increases nausea and vomiting which is not reduced by adding droperidol.[21]

- Midazolam 0.5 mg/kg orally in orange squash.

Shivering

Postoperative shivering is relieved by pethidine 20 mg IV. Orphenadrine 50 mg po (IV is not easily available in UK) or procyclidine 5 to 10 mg IV is suggested as being better than methylphenidate for postoperative rigidity and shivering on the grounds of being less addictive.[22]

Steroid therapy perioperatively[2,23]

Trauma and major surgery increase cortisol secretion from 30 mg/day to 75–150 mg/day. A patient taking regular corticosteroid therapy may have a suppressed hypothalamic–pituitary–adrenal axis (HPA). HPA suppression can occur with as little as 1.5 mg/day of inhaled beclomethasone, or a week of oral therapy. Some recommended regimes probably give an excess of steroid supplements for the average patient receiving steroids.

Perioperative steroid regime

> *Minor/day surgery*
> Continue normal oral steroid therapy.
> *Moderate or major surgery or trauma*
> Preoperatively take normal oral steroid dose.
> During surgery – Hydrocortisone 25 mg IV at induction and 100 mg/24 h for 24 h postoperatively after moderate surgery and for 48–72 h or until starting oral therapy after major surgery (Hydrocortisone 20 mg = prednisolone 5 mg).

Patient taking higher doses of prednisolone e.g. 40 mg, should have the amount of hydrocortisone doubled.

Patient taking high doses of steroid for immunosupression should have their prednisolone replaced by an equivalent dose of hydrocortisone IV until able to take oral drugs.

Addison's disease patients, with no functioning pituitary or adrenal glands, require continuous steroid therapy of hydrocortisone 20–30 mg/day with fludrocortisone 50–300 μg. Monitoring should include: conscious level (drowsiness may indicate a lack of steroid), blood glucose, sodium and potassium. During surgery additional hydrocortisone should be given as for major surgery.

More hydrocortisone should be considered in any patient who becomes drowsy or has abnormal electrolytes.

Hydrocortisone IV should also be given to resuscitate an acute hypothyroid or myxoedema crisis.

Suxamethonium apnoea

A dose of 1–1.5 mg/kg normally causes paralysis for up to 5 min. Paralysis is prolonged when serum cholinesterase is deficient or absent. This occurs for a short time in pregnancy around the time of delivery, liver disease, plasmapheresis and genetic deficiency in the production of the normal enzyme. Heterozygotes produce some normal enzyme and may have a prolonged action for up to 20 min. Homozygotes will hydrolyse suxamethonium slowly by other enzymes taking 2–4 h.

If a patient fails to recover neuromuscular function within 15 min after suxamethonium they probably suffer from a deficiency of cholinesterase.

Management of prolonged neuromuscular block

- Oxygenate by intubation or laryngeal mask and ventilate.

- Unaware by continuing with anaesthetic agents or IV drugs such as midazolam and propofol.

- Monitor vital signs and response to nerve stimulator.

- Allow time for full recovery of skeletal muscle function. Do not extubate at the first sign of returning power. The diaphragm recovers before other skeletal muscles.

- Intravenous crystalloid infusion 10–20 ml/kg increases the volume for distribution and increases renal excretion.

- Take serum for cholinesterase assay.

- Later, interview blood relatives and screen for cholinesterase levels.

- Give the results in writing to patient and GP. Consider an alert bracelet.

Suxamethonium pain

- A small dose of a non depolarising muscle relaxant (atracurium 7 mg IV) given 2 min before suxamethonium will reduce the pain.

- Lysine acetyl salicylate 13 mg/kg IV given 3 min before the administration of suxamethonium reduced the incidence and intensity of suxamethonium induced myalgia. Other prostaglandin inhibitors should be equally effective.[24]

Tetanus

- Baclofen 1000 µg for patients between 16 and 55 years, 800 µg over 55 years and 500 µg under 16 years was given intrathecally. This relieves spasm for 24–48 h in milder cases but may cause respiratory depression. Flumazenil may reverse this respiratory depression[25].

- Baclofen 600–800 µg/day, intrathecally by continuous infusion may relieve spasticity and enable weaning from the ventilator.[26]

- Dantolene has been used to control painful muscle spasms and trismus in patients with less severe tetanus and is more effective than a benzodiazepine. A dose of 0.5–1 mg/kg IV repeated every 6 h if necessary is recommended.[27]

References

1. Alberti KGMM, Thomas RJB. The management of diabetes during surgery. *British Journal of Anaesthesia* 1979; **51**: 693–710.

69

Drugs

D

2. Drugs in the peri-operative period. *Drugs and Therapeutics Bulletin* 1999; **37:** 68–70.
3. Hall GM, Desborough JP. Diabetes and anaesthesia – slow progress? *Anaesthesia* 1988; **43:** 531–2.
4. Christiansen CL, Schurizeck BA, Malling B, Knudsen L, Alberti KGMM, Hermansen K. Insulin treatment for insulin-dependent diabetic patients undergoing minor surgery. *Anaesthesia* 1988; **43:** 533–7.
5. Maitre PO, Shafer SL. A simple pocket calculator approach to predict anesthetic drug concentrations from pharmacokinetic data. *Anesthesiology* 1990; **73:** 332–6.
6. McKiernan EP. An even simpler way to determine drug infusion rates. *Anesthesiology* 1985; **63:** 459–60.
7. Sherry E, Burton GW, Wilkins DG. Infusion nomograms. *Anaesthesia* 1993; **48:** 396–401.
8. Wood M. Erythromycin inhibits the metabolism of theophylline, alfentanyl, midazolam and erythromycin. *British Journal of Anaesthesia* 1990; **65:** 131.
9. Bretschneider H. Osmolarity of commercially supplied drugs often used in anesthesia. *Anesthesia and Analgesia* 1987; **66:** 361–2.
10. Kishikawa K et al. Diltiazem for ventricular fibrillation. *Anesthesiology* 1997; **87:** 709.
11. Bannon MG. Termination of hiccups occurring under anesthesia. *Anesthesiology* 1991; **74:** 385.
12. Saitto C, Gristina G, Cosmi EV. Treatment of hiccups by continuous positive airway pressure (CPAP) in anesthetised subjects. *Anesthesiology* 1982; **57:** 345.
13. Beerle BJ, Arriaga M. Myringotomy tube placement – another role for EMLA cream. *Anesthesia and Analgesia* 1996; **83:** 435.
14. Bruce DL. MAC values of mixtures. *Anesthesiology* 1983; **59:** 599.
15. Kobin DD et al. Minimum alveolar concentrations and oil/gas partition coefficients of four anaesthetic isomers. *Anesthesiology* 1981; **54:** 314–17.
16. Sydow M, Radke J. High dose intravenous magnesium sulphate in the management of life threatening status asthmaticus. *Intensive Care Medicine* 1995; **21:** 94–5.
17. Gorchein A. Drug treatment in acute porphyria. *British Journal of Pharmacology* 1997; **44:** 427–34.
18. Ashley EM. Anaesthesia for porphyria. *British Journal of Hospital Medicine* 1996; **56:** 37–42.
19. Elcock D, Norris A. Elevated porphoryns following proprofol anaesthesia in acute intermttent porphyria. *Anaesthesia* 1994; **49:** 957–8.
20. Gutstein HB, Johnson KL, Heard MB, Gregory GA. Oral ketamine preanaesthetic medication for children. *Anesthesiology* 1992; **76:** 28–33.
21. Friessen RH, Lockhart CH. Oral transmucosal fentanyl citrate for preanaesthetic medication of paediatric day surgery patients with and without droperidol as a prophylactic anti-emetic. *Anaesthesia* 1992; **76:** 46–51.
22. Fry ENS. Postoperative shivering. *Anaesthesia* 1983; **38:** 172.
23. Nicholson G, Burrin JM, Hall GM. Peri-operative steroid supplementation. *Anaesthesia* 1998; **53:** 1091–104.
24. Naguib M. Prostaglandin inhibitors and suxamethonium induced myalgia. *British Journal of Anaesthesia* 1994; **72:** 139–40.
25. Saissy JM et al. Treatment of severe tetanus by intrathecal injections of baclofen without artificial ventilation. *Intensive Care Medicine* 1992; **18:** 241–4.
26. Pellanda A, Caldiroli D, Vaghi GM, Bonelli. Treatment of severe tetanus by intrathecal infusion of baclofen. *Intensive Care Medicine* 1993; **60:** 59.
27. Sternlo JE, Andersen LW. Early treatment of mild tetanus with dantrolene. *Intensive Care Medicine* 1990; **16:** 345.

Drugs

D

ECG

A 12 lead ECG is obtained from

- Lead I: right arm to left arm.
- Lead II: right arm to left leg.
- Lead III: left arm to left leg.
- AVR – right arm to left arm and left leg.
- AVL – left arm to right arm and left leg.
- AVF – left leg to right arm and left arm.
- Chest leads V 1–6.

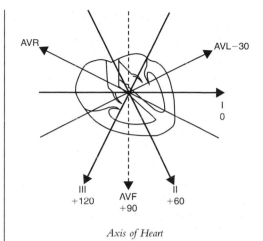

Axis of Heart

Calibration

- 1 cm vertical = 1 mV.
- 0.5 cm horizontal = 0.2 s
- Rate: There are 300 squares of 0.2 s in 1 min (300×0.2 s = 60 s). So if the rate is regular, divide 300 by the number of large squares between two consecutive R waves to give the rate per minute. If the rate is irregular take a number of beats (y) and count the total number of squares from the first R wave to the last R wave then 300×y divided by number of squares = rate/min.

Axis

- Consider a circle with 0° at 3 o'clock. Then the normal axis is from −30 to +90. AVL −30°, lead I 0°, lead II 60°, AVF 90°, lead III 120°, AVR 150°.
- To determine the heart axis look for the lead with the maximum positive deflection. This will give the line of the axis. Or take the lead with equal positive and negative deflections. The axis will lie at right angles to this lead.

Rhythm

- Supraventricular dysrhythmias: look for P waves and their association to the QRS which should be narrow in time.
- Regularity of QRS complex. Ventricular dysrhythmias give wide and abnormal QRS complexes.
- Identify: atrial flutter, fibrillation, heart block – first degree with PR over 0.2 s, second degree with dropped beats or some Ps linked to QRS, third degree complete block QRS rate of 30/min.

P wave

- Right atrial enlargement; tall and peaked, P pulmonale.
- Left atrial enlargement; bifid in shape of M, P mitrale.

Ischaemia

- ST segment depressed >1 mm, inverted or tall pointed T waves.

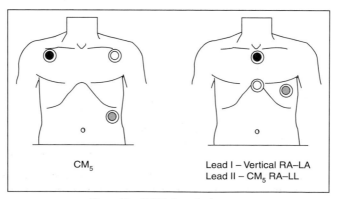

Myocardial infarction

Q wave broad >1 mm, deep >2 mm (abnormal Q in AVR, V1, LBBB, Wolff Parkinson–White syndrome).

Infarction shows in leads facing the infarct so:

- Inferior wall in II, III, AVF.
- Lateral wall in I, II, AVL.
- Anterior wall in V2 to V5.

Wolff Parkinson–White syndrome

- Wide QRS begins with a slurred delta waves, J wave, short PR interval.

Left ventricular hypertrophy

- Left axis. Add deepest Q in V1 or V2 to tallest R in V4 or V5 to give >35 cm.

Right heart strain and pulmonary embolism

- Right axis, RBBB, T inverted in V1 and V2, sometimes S lead II with Q and inverted T in III, lack of progression through V1 to V5.

Digoxin therapy gives a depressed ST segment in the shape of a reversed tick.

Three lead electrode position

The CM₅ configuration is the bipolar equivalent of V5 which shows nearly 90% of all S–T segment changes (Figure 18).

Lead II is best for dysrhythmia detection because of the large P wave.

V1 is best for bundle branch block and differentiation of right from left ventricular ectopics.

- All three configurations can be obtained by placing electrodes at the manubrium sterni (RA), xiphisternum (LA) and at V5 position (LL). Lead II (RA–LL), equivalent to CM₅ gives good detection of ischaemia, while lead I (RA–LA), now vertical – manubrium to xiphisternum, gives maximum P waves with amplitudes a little less than an oesophageal lead.

- The incidence of muscle and respiratory artefacts is low.[1]

A reduction in the amplitude of the ECG complexes may be a sign of reduced cardiac output or of a pneumothorax.

- Leads over the left side of chest with a left pneumothorax will show a greater reduction than in a right sided

CM₅

Lead I – Vertical RA–LA
Lead II – CM₅ RA–LL

Figure 18 – ECG electrode placements.

pneumothorax. If the patient is having surgery or has suffered trauma to one side of the chest it may be useful to place the ECG electrodes over that side to be more likely to detect a pneumothorax.[2]

The diagnosis of dysrhythmias can be difficult in the presence of a tachycardia.

- The oesophageal lead often augments the P wave. An oesophageal lead can be made from an intravascular J wire placed inside a small diameter catheter so that only the last 3 mm flexible part protrudes beyond the end of the catheter.[3]

Education

- A number of line diagrams may make it easier for the anaesthetist to explain a procedure and easier for patients to understand the nature of the problem.[4] (Figure 19).

Elderly and Anaesthesia

Avoid hypoxia and hypotension:

- P_aO_2 falls with age = P_aO_2 − age/3 mmHg.
- cerebral blood flow = $59 - (0.3 \times age)$ ml/100 g/min.

Drugs

Give smaller first dose because effect potentiated by

- reduced number of receptor sites,
- reduced body water and reduced plasma proteins lead to a higher plasma concentration.

Give repeat doses less often as drug effect prolonged due to

- reduced renal excretion and reduced liver metabolism.

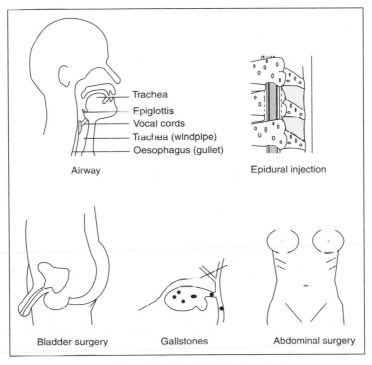

Trachea
Epiglottis
Vocal cords
Trachea (windpipe)
Oesophagus (gullet)

Airway

Epidural injection

Bladder surgery

Gallstones

Abdominal surgery

Figure 19 – Educational drawings.

Elderly system changes

System	Changes
Tissues	Less body water, reduced muscle mass, bones brittle, kyphoscoliosis, calcified ligaments
CNS	Reduced cell and receptor mass, easily confused. Reduced hearing, and vision
RS	Low compliance, higher closing volume within TV, loss of alveoli, impaired coughing, prone to hypoxia
CVS	Reduced muscle contractility, ischaemia, delayed conduction
Renal	Reduced concentrating capacity
Liver	Reduced enzyme activity
Blood	Reduced blood volume, reduced red cell mass, bruise more easily
Endocrine	Possible diabetes, hypothyroid, reduced endocrine production
At risk from	Cooling, tissue and nerve damage

References

1. Wicks M, Hunt J, Walker R, Torda TA. An electrode montage for electrocardiographic monitoring. *Anaesthesia and Intensive Care* 1989; **17:** 74–7.
2. Brocke-Utne JG, Botz G. Are electrocardiographic changes the first sign of impending peri-operative pneumothorax? *Anaesthesia* 1993; **48:** 543–4.
3. Brown DL, Greenberg DJ. A simple device for monitoring the oesophageal electrocardiogram. *Anesthesiology* 1983; **59:** 482–3.
4. Birkinshaw K. Pre-operative approaches to patients. *Anaesthesia* 1978; **33:** 483–7.

Fasting

Prolonged fasting leads to an increase in: gastric secretions, acidity of the secretions, abdominal discomfort, dehydration and hypoglycaemia, especially in children. In elective cases it is suggested that clear fluids – water, squash, tea or coffee should be taken up to 2 h preoperatively.[1-3]

Give	Effect
5–10 ml/kg water, squash, tea or coffee up to 2 h before procedure	Reduces gastric fluid volume, raises pH
	Maintains hydration
Not a food drink e.g. milk	Prevents hypoglycaemia
Orange juice is said to increase stomach acidity	Prevents abdominal pain
Added glucose in children	Aids early mobilisation
Food up to 6 h before procedure	

References

1. Goresky GV, Maltby JR. Fasting guidelines for elective surgical procedures. *Canadian Journal of Anaesthesiology* 1990; **37:** 493–5.
2. Read MS, Vaughan RS. Allowing preoperative patients to drink, effect on patients' safety and comfort of unlimited oral water until 2 h before anaesthesia. *Acta Anesthesiologica Scandinavia* 1991; **35:** 591–5.
3. Strunin L. How long should patients fast before surgery? Time for new guidelines. *Anaesthesia* 1993; **70:** 1–3.

Forceps

The usefulness of the Magill forceps can be improved by

- Bending the distal arms twice to conform to the oropharynx[1] or just curved to match the shape of the Macintosh laryngoscope.[2]

- Rounding the ends outwardly to give a smooth surface to the mucosa and the arms bent in the sagittal plane to give a forward concavity. This better fits the shape of the pharynx for assisted intubation.[3]

- The distal ends modified so that one side has two prongs and the other a single prong which comes to the centre of the two pronged side. This arrangement improves the grip.[4]

References

1. Rees DF. A modification of Magill's forceps. *Anaesthesia* 1976; **31:** 302–3.
2. Nott MR. Modified Magill's forceps. *Anaesthesia* 1996; **51:** 612.
3. Agosti L. Modification of Magill's intubating forceps. *Anaesthesia* 1976; **31:** 574.
4. Pelimon A, Simunovic Z. Modified Magill forceps for difficult tracheal intubation. *Anaesthesia* 1987; **42:** 83.

Infection Control

Procedure for treating and limiting exposure to body fluids that could be contaminated with human immunodeficiency virus (HIV), hepatitis B virus (HBV) and hepatitis C virus (HCV).

Treatment

Sharp injuries, needle-stick and cuts:

- squeeze wound to bleed, do not scrub,
- wash wound with soap and running water,
- apply dressing.

Splashes of fluid to broken skin (e.g. cuts, eczema), mucous membranes of eyes or mouth:

- wash area with large amounts of water,
- wash eyes before and after removing contact lenses, refer to eye department Document incident.

If the patient could be an unconfirmed source of HIV, HBC, HCV:

- Ask patient's consent for blood sample to be taken.
- The result should be given in confidence to the patient.
- Make telephone contact with laboratory and arrange urgent analysis.

If positive result or patient refuses, treat as positive

- HIV: Post-exposure prophylaxis as soon as possible after exposure.
- HBC: Booster vaccination if blood shows low antibody levels.
- HCV: No prevention available.

Management of patient with HIV disease

- The patient must give informed consent, preferably written, before serological testing for antibodies to HIV.

- It cannot be assumed that a patient is free from HIV infection when there is a negative test for antibodies.
- Hand washing before and after contact is the most important means of preventing cross infection.
- Masks and eye protection should be worn whenever a procedure involving blood or body fluids is likely to cause splashes.
- All specimens must be labelled as "Danger of Infection" and sealed.
- To prevent needle-stick injury wear disposable gloves and plastic apron. Dispose of needles and sharps directly into a rigid leak proof sharps container, which is kept near to the site of injection.
- Do not leave any sharp lying about.
- Do not try to reinsert a sharp into its container.
- Consider alternative means of injection including no needle techniques.
- All instruments should be placed in marked bags without washing and either disposed of or returned to a sterilisation department.
- Spills should be cleared by staff wearing gloves and plastic apron. Wipe with disposable paper towels and NaDCC solution made to 10,000 ppm available chlorine. 7×2.5 g tablets in 1 l water.

When a procedure involving opening the skin is to be carried out e.g. operation, drain, dressing change

- remove all unnecessary equipment from the area;
- all staff should wear disposable gloves, mask over eyes and mouth, plastic aprons

and do not leave the area without removing these into marked bags;

- inform other departments beforehand that a specimen is being sent;

- spills of body fluid and all equipment should be wiped with disposable cloths and NaDCC solution and allowed to dry.

Critical care and antibiotics (Table 4)

Diagnosis of infection based on

1. pyrexia, rising CRP, rising WCC;

2. screen for source of sepsis:

   - blood culture from peripheral vein and central lines;

   - tracheal aspirate, urine MSU or catheter, CRP, wound swabs;

   - serology for atypical organisms: urine for Legionella antigen.

3. CRP, CK.

Consider imaging abdomen ultrasound or CT, sinus X-ray.

Interosseous Needle when venous access is difficult

- Particularly in children, multiple trauma and burnt patients.

- An interosseous needle can be placed into the medial surface of the tibia, 2 cm above the medial malleolus or 1–2 cm below and medial to the tibial tuberosity. The skin is cleaned, local anaesthetic infiltrated subcutaneously and the needle screwed, not pushed, through the cortex and then advanced a further 2–3 cm (Figure 20).

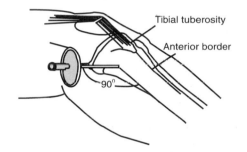

Figure 20 – Interosseous cannulation.

Table 4 – Critical care antibiotics

Infection	Therapy IV
Respiratory infection	
Community acquired	British Thoracic Society guidelines Erythromycin + Cefotaxime
Hospital acquired >48 h stay	Cefotaxime ± Teicoplanin Levofloxacin
Acquired in ITU	Imipenem or Levofloxacin + Teicoplanin
Aspiration pneumonia	Cefotaxime + Metronidazole
Infections associated with abdominal surgery	Amoxycillin 1 2 g tds I Gentamycin 4 mg/kg once daily I Metronidazole 500 mg tds
Line associated infection	If line is >3 days old, replace if possible at a different site with Teicoplanin cover. If line is precious, quantitative blood cultures to confirm infection.
	As a last resort replace line over a guided wire under Teicoplanin cover.
Meningitis	Cefotaxime + Benzylpenicillin, add Rifampicin if *Streptococcus pneumoniae* is a possibility if patient is "in extremis".

Dr Cefai, Microbiologist.

- In the correct position the needle will stay upright without support. Blood or marrow is aspirated if possible and injection does not produce a swelling in surrounding tissues.

- Fluids, blood and drugs have to be administered under pressure until an alternative vascular route can be established. Firm fixation with material such as plaster of Paris is essential.[1,2]

References

1. Alba RM, Lopez MJR, Flores JC. Use of the interosseous route in resuscitation. *Intensive Care Medicine* 1994; **20:** 529.
2. Stewart FC, Kain ZN. Intraosseous infusion: elective use in paediatric anesthesia. *Anesthesia and Analgesia* 1992; **75:** 626–9.

Inspiratory Stridor

Inspiratory Stridor means upper airway obstruction.

Treatment: clear airway, forward thrust of mandible, Guedel or nasal airway, 100% oxygen and sit up.

Laryngeal oedema found with

- previous recent intubation,

- laryngitis,

- anaphylactic reactions,

- a large weight gain in pregnancy and pre-eclampsia syndrome at term.[1]

Treatment: humidified oxygen, intubation, treat cause.

Laryngospasm

Postoperatively and when the larynx is hyperexcitable.

- Treatment: 100% humidified oxygen and sit up.

- Midazolam 5–10 mg IV.

- Diazemules 5–10 mg IV.

- Lidocaine spray 10 mg × 5 to larynx, best as a prophylactic measure in at risk patients e.g. before extubation following a laryngeal biopsy.

- Extreme state: IV induction agent, suxamethonium and intubation.

Jehovah's Witnesses

Close cooperation with the patient is essential to determine what is acceptable. If in doubt an elder can be contacted 020 8906 2211.

- An advanced medical directive or other written and signed consent form must be respected as the wishes of the patient. Hospitals should have specific forms.

- Most believers will not accept a transfusion of whole blood or any blood products such as fresh frozen plasma.

- Children below the age of consent may be able to give consent. The "Gillick-competence" ruling suggested that below 12 years the child is not able to understand the nature of consent. Children should be treated on the grounds that the child's well being is paramount. If blood is to be administered then a "Specific Issue Order" may be required from the High Court. In Scotland application is made under Section 11 of the Children Act 1995. In a life threatening emergency, in a child, blood should be given to save life and the consent of the court taken afterwards.

All steps should be taken to limit blood loss by position, hypotensive technique, tourniquet, vasoconstictors and haemodilution, careful surgical technique and haemostasis. A cell saver may be acceptable and tranexanic acid or aprotinin given to reduce fibrinolysis.

Elective cases may be transferred to hospital teams prepared to undertake such surgery as advised by the patient.

At all times consultant staff must be involved. All discussions with the patient should be in an open and in non-judgemental way. Decisions should be documented in the notes.

See: Management of Anaesthesia for Jehovah's Witnesses. Association of Anaesthetists of Great Britain and Ireland, March 1999.

Latex Allergy[2]

Identify patients at risk:

- Health care workers with repeated use of latex gloves, repeated bladder catheterisation, multiple operations, cross allergy with bananas, avocados, kiwi fruits, allergies or contact dermatitis of uncertain origin occurring during previous surgery.

- Itch, swelling or redness after contact with rubber.

- Swelling of tongue with dental treatment or blowing balloons.

Preoperatively consider giving IV:

- chlorpheniramine 10 mg (0.25 mg/kg),

- ranitidine 50 mg (1 mg/kg),

- hydrocortisone 100 mg (2 mg/kg); repeat every 6–8 h.

Operation

Use a theatre which has been unoccupied for at least 2 h to reduce the level of aerosolised latex antigens.

Make a latex free box which contains:[2]

- Database of latex free equipment.

- List of latex containing equipment to be avoided.

- List of latex containing equipment that can be used with precautions.

Appropriate treatment for use with allergic patient

- includes latex free gloves (not just hypoallergenic);

- avoids rubber IV bungs;

- includes latex free syringes.

Local Anaesthesia

Local anaesthetic blocks

Before any local anaesthetic block is performed

- Obtain the patient's informed consent, particularly if there is a chronic neurological disease such as multiple sclerosis.

- Check there is no disturbance of coagulation.

- No infection at the site of block.

- Know the anatomy of the site.

- Check the equipment, use a nerve stimulator.

- Establish IV access in case of an intravascular injection of LA and monitor for hypotension and level of consciousness.

- Treat hypotension with an alpha and beta agonist and IV fluid. Treat loss of consciousness and seizure by protecting the airway and IPPV, but care to maintain cardiac output.

- Resuscitation equipment and drugs for hypotension and seizures.

Short bevel needle

Needle design for nerve block

- Short bevelled needles are less likely to enter nerve fascicles. If the needle becomes intrafascicular with fascicular impalement then long bevelled needles and perhaps pencil point needles are less traumatic. It is possible to prevent intrafascicular needle placement by using a high quality nerve stimulator which gives the range of current 0.2–0.5 mA (see nerve stimulators). Much smaller currents are required to stimulate axons from an intrafascicular, than an extrafascicular electrode. When needles impale fascicules paraesthesia will occur and some 10% of patients will have persistent paraesthesia for days, but serious prolonged complications are rare.[3]

- To aid the passage of such local block needles the epidermis and dermis can first be broken with a blood lancet.[4]

Sensory testing

- A variety of pointers have been used to test the effect of local anaesthesia but it is desirable not to produce scratches or other skin damage.

- Wipe the skin with an alcohol/spirit antiseptic swab. As it evaporates cold is felt in normal skin. Cold from a metal stethoscope and pressure is also used.

- An open safety pin pushed through a rubber stopper with 5 mm protruding will give a sensation of pin prick without pain. The other end of the pin can be used to test for pressure. A new pin should be used for each patient[5] (Figure 21).

Sensitivity is improved by

- The use of the smallest gauge needle, attached to a length of extension tubing, increases the fingers' appreciation of the feel of the needle passing through tissue planes. As the fine needle is advanced it may be felt to go though the fibrous sheath, which surrounds the brachial plexus.

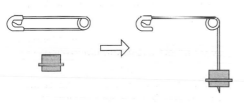
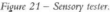

Figure 21 – Sensory tester.

- When the needle breaks through the fibrous sheath of the perivascular interscalene space a click is felt. Local anaesthetic (LA) solution of 1 or 2 ml is injected and the syringe removed. A few drops of solution will flow back and fall from the needle hub. This is due to an increase in pressure inside the space. If the fluid is outside the space no flow back is seen.[6]

Head and Neck

Supraorbital and supratrochlear nerves

- Use: Incisions of the scalp anterior to the crown.

- Block: The supraorbital nerve emerges from a notch in the mid–superior margin of the orbit 2–3 cm from the medial end. The trochlear nerve lies 1 cm medially. Up to 5 ml of LA with adrenaline are infiltrated on both sides, just above the medial half of the superior margin of the orbit.

- Produces anaesthesia of the scalp back to the crown.

Eye

- Use. Eye surgery.

- Blocks: periorbital or peribulbar – needle not introduced past the length of the eye; retrobulbar – needle introduced past the length of the orbit either outside or inside the cone of muscles.

- Two problems to avoid: penetrating the eye ball and damaging the optic nerve.

- Eye ball penetration: A blunt pointed needle is less likely to puncture the sclera but is more painful to inject than a sharp pointed needle. Avoid puncturing the sclera by using a gentle approach; the eye should not move when the needle moves and visa versa. The sclera is extremely tough and difficult to puncture without force.

- Optic nerve. If the needle does not penetrate more than the depth of the eye it cannot damage the optic nerve. The eye has an axial length of 20–25 mm, except in myopic eyes, when it is longer. Once a needle penetrates more than 25 mm from the front of the eye it must be retrobulbar and can damage the optic nerve. Using the inferior lateral approach a needle injected more than 25 mm may be retrobulbar, in or outside the cone. The optic nerve lies medial in the orbit so a needle injected using a superior medial approach should only be injected for 10–12 mm.

- Other complications: Haemtoma leads to proptosis, apply pressure. Subarachnoid block, if too deep, and intravascular injection require urgent resuscitation. Subconjunctival oedema (chemosis) is common. Corneal abrasion.

- Various mixtures of local anaesthetic are used including 2% lidocaine with 1 : 400 000 adrenaline, 2% lidocaine and 0.5% bupivacaine in equal volumes to 12–15 ml. Hyaluronidase 500 unit is added to increase spread.

Technique

- A periocular or peribulbar block is performed with the patient supine and looking straight ahead so that the optic nerve lies on the medial side of the sagittal plane.

- The conjunctiva is anaesthetised with increasing concentrations of local anaesthetic.

- A 25G needle is passed from the infero-lateral angle of the orbit, through the conjunctiva or lower eyelid along the floor of the orbit to a depth of no more than 25 mm, depending on the diameter of the eyeball, to avoid the optic nerve. A give is felt as it passes through the lower lateral septum. The eye ball should not move

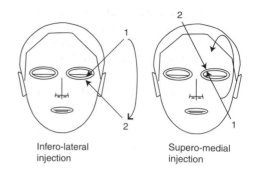

| Infero-lateral injection | Supero-medial injection |

Figure 22 – Local anaesthesia for eye surgery.

when the needle is moved. The patient looks straight ahead. After aspiration 3–5 ml LA are injected without pain or resistance. In many patients, at the inferio-lateral part of the fibromuscular cone there is a deficit making a communication between the space outside and inside the cone. The patient should probably not move the eye to look medially as this will bring the optic nerve towards the needle. As the needle is withdrawn 1–2 ml is injected into orbicularis oculi muscle (Figure 22).

- If the needle is passed in more than 25 mm from the front of the eye it is retrobulbar. If outside the cone it is pericone. If it is then passed upwards it will become inside the cone – intracone, with risk of optic nerve damage. It is possible to make an intraconal injection which is not strictly behind the globe and so not retrobulbar. The advantage of the intraconal injection is that it rapidly blocks the sensory nerves of the eye which are all within the cone.

- A second injection superio-medially may be needed. The medial injection increases LA spread to the motor supply of the superior oblique muscle, which is attached to the superior aspect of the globe and runs medially, and to the orbicularis muscle.[7] A 25G needle is introduced superio-medially through the upper lid or conjunctiva aimed at the roof of the orbit, parallel to the nose to a depth of 10–12 mm, 2–3 ml of LA are injected. Another 1 ml is injected on withdrawal into the muscle. In the elderly poor orbital septa may allow LA to leak into the eyelid and a larger volume of LA may be required.[8]

- It is suggested that the needle should be inserted with a 5° nasal direction away from the sagittal plane in order to avoid injecting into the medial rectus muscle giving myotoxicity.

- A few patients experience pain with the single injection due to the nasociliary nerve which carries corneal and circumcorneal pain sensation, being within the cone of muscles. It may escape block by a peribulbar injection.

- The approaches using intraconal and medial peribulbar injections achieve a rapid onset of globe and lid akinesia and patient comfort.[9]

- A single injection, medial peribulbar approach using 8 ml of 3% prilocaine "fills" both upper and lower eyelids. If halfway through injection, one eyelid is not filling, the needle is withdrawn and re-inserted inclined slightly towards the unfilled eyelid.[10,11]

Glossopharyngeal nerve

- Use. A bilateral glossopharyngeal block reduces gagging during awake fibre-optic intubation.

- The lingular branch passes from the lower border of the superior constrictor and enters the submucosa near the base of the posterior tonsillar pillar. Local anaesthetic injected at the base of the tonsillar pillar should spread to the lingual branch. The tongue is displaced to the opposite side and a 25G needle inserted to 0.5 cm deep

just lateral to the base of the anterior tonsillar pillar; 2 ml LA is injected on each side.[12]

- Another technique applies topical anaesthetic to the mucosa of the pillar area.

Long thoracic nerve

- Use. Patients with intractable pain in the chest wall may have pain from serratus anterior muscle spasm supplied by the long thoracic nerve (Figure 23).

- The long thoracic nerve is blocked in the neck, posterior to the brachial plexus and anterior to the eleventh cranial nerve.

- The patient is supine and the middle scalene muscle is identified by palpating or rolling the index and middle fingers laterally, and feeling from in-front backwards, sternomastoid, scalenus anterior, the interscalene grove and then the middle scalene muscle. A 22G needle, attached to a nerve stimulator, is advanced through the middle scalene muscle from slightly above the level of C6 directed caudally and slightly laterally, parallel to the long axis of the middle scalene muscle. If trapezius contracts then the spinal accessory muscle has been stimulated and the needle is redirected more anteriorly until serratus anterior contracts. If the brachial plexus is stimulated the needle should be redirected posteriorly. When the nerve is blocked the

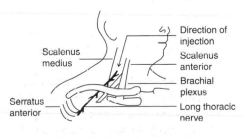

Figure 23   Long thoracic nerve.

arm cannot be abducted beyond 90° and the scapula wings. If the serratus anterior is stimulated in the course of a brachial plexus block the needle should be redirected more anteriorly.[13]

Superficial cervical plexus block

- Use. Procedures on the anterior neck including cannulation of the internal jugular vein, subclavian vein with suturing, incisions above the clavicles and analgesia for the insertion of a catheter under the clavicle.[14] Pain relief for thyroidectomy.

- The plexus becomes superficial at the mid-point of the posterior border of sternomastoid. A 25G 30 mm needle is inserted at this mid-point and 5–10 ml of LA is infiltrated to a depth of 3–4 cm, in a fanwise direction, cephalad and caudally along the posterior edge of the muscle.

Suprascapular nerve block

- Use. Management of painful shoulder conditions: frozen shoulder,[15] cancer head of the humerus (longer block with cryolesions[16]) and postoperative shoulder pain[17] (Figures 24 and 25).

- The classical method is to bisect the scapular angle. But the spine is easier to feel

than the angle. Using a nerve stimulator, look for supraspinatus or infraspinatus twitch and the assistant will feel abduction and external rotation of the arm.

- Ten ml of 0.25% bupivacaine is injected one-finger breadth superior to the mid-point of the spine of the scapular. Paraesthesia is sought 3–4 cm from the surface of the skin. The scapula should be elevated away from the posterior chest wall by flexing the arm at the elbow and rotating medially so that the hand is placed on the opposite shoulder. This should reduce the possibility of producing a pneumothorax, especially in thin patients.[18]

- Another landmark is obtained by drawing a line along the length of the scapula spine and dividing it into thirds, a second line

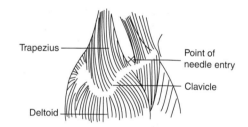

Figure 25 – Antero-lateral view of shoulder showing point of injection for suprascapular nerve block at junction of trapezius muscle with clavicle.

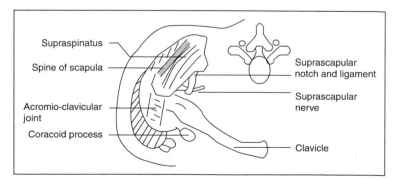

Figure 24 – Superior view of shoulder showing relationship of suprascapular nerve to clavicle.

is drawn perpendicular to the first at the junction of the medial third and lateral two-thirds. The scapular notch lies 1–2 cm cranial to the point of intersection. The needle is inserted at this later point and the nerve is found at a depth of 1.5–3 cm.

Brachial plexus block

Interscalene approach

The brachial plexus is formed from the anterior primary rami of C5 to T1 nerve roots. An even block is obtained if entry is into the mid-point of the plexus and not too high. Entry below C7 increases the risk of pneumothorax.

- The optimum point for needle entry is found by passing a stimulating electrode over the skin from the posterior edge of the sternocleidomastoid (SCM) laterally to the middle of the posterior triangle of the neck. The needle is inserted where the best contraction of deltoid, biceps or brachial radialis is obtained with a current under 0.5 mA. The skin electrode is made from an ECG electrode trimmed to 0.5 cm in diameter attached to the cathode of a nerve stimulator set at 2–5 mA.[19]

- The interscalene grove is made prominent by asking the patient to take a deep inspiration against a closed mouth and nose.

- Another landmark for needle entry into the interscalene groove starts with the head turned to the opposite side. A line is drawn from the apex of the division of SCM to the most medial insertion of the trapezius muscle on the clavicle. The needle is inserted at the point where the external jugular vein crosses this line.

- When the anatomy makes it difficult to palpate the interscalene grove a line is drawn laterally at C6 (cricoid cartilage

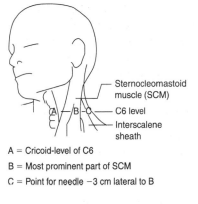

A = Cricoid-level of C6
B = Most prominent part of SCM
C = Point for needle −3 cm lateral to B

Figure 26 – Interscalene block.

or Chassanac's tubercle). A point, on this line, 3 cm posteriorly from the most prominent part of the belly of sternomastoid at the level of C6 will give the point for a needle to enter the grove[20] (Figure 26).

- The deltoid muscle is innervated by the axillary nerve which arises from C5 and C6 roots. The primary nerves supplying the shoulder joint and surrounding muscles are also supplied by the same roots. The inability to abduct the upper arm using the deltoid muscle is a 100% indicator of a successful interscalene block for shoulder procedures.[21]

Supraclavicular block

The subclavian artery is palpated as it passes over the first rib behind the mid-point of the clavicle. With a finger on the artery a needle is introduced behind the artery backwards towards the first rib in the line of the nipple, feeling for a click as the nerve sheath is entered. Once the depth of the rib is felt the needle is walked posteriorly or anteriorly until paraesthesia is obtained. There is no need to move the needle medially where it will walk off the rib and into the pleura to give a pneumothorax.

- The effectiveness of a brachial plexus block depends on the distribution of the paraesthesia evoked by a nerve stimulator. In performing a supraclavicular block if paraesthesia is in the distribution of the median nerve then success is greater than when it is in the distribution of the ulnar or radial nerves. It is suggested that the median nerve represents the anterior division of the middle trunk.[22] Paraesthesia in the middle trunk gives the greatest success.[23] The middle trunk is more central anatomically for the distribution of the LA.

Subclavicular perivascular block

Alternative but similar to a supraclavicular block.

Landmarks – subclavian artery as it passes over the first rib and the interscalene grove. The needle is introduced behind the subclavian artery into the interscalene grove, more posterior and medial than in a supraclavicular block. The needle is directed caudally. The injection is made after a click is felt as the sheath is entered and paraesthesia is induced in the hands.

Axillary block

The axillary artery lies between coracobrachialis anteriorly and teres minor posteriorly.

- The arm is abducted to 90° with the hand resting on the pillow next to the head of the patient. A 10 ml syringe, filled with normal saline, is attached to a 22G × 51mm cannula. The operator's index finger is pressed over the axillary artery as near to the anterior axillary fold as possible. The needle is inserted below the index finger at 20° to the skin. The needle is advanced parallel to the artery and continuous pressure is applied to the syringe plunger until loss of resistance is found. An aspiration test is made before injecting 30 ml of LA.[24]

- The axillary artery can be brought into prominence by applying an arterial tourniquet to the upper arm which is then abducted to 90°. The artery in the axilla is distended and the pulse bounding. The advancing needle feels the wall of the artery as tapping. Winnie has shown that the tourniquet will not compress the axillary sheath to limit LA flow.[25]

- The axillary artery may be difficult to palpate. The exploring finger presses in the axilla while the radial artery is palpated or the pulse oximeter signal is observed. When the axillary artery is compressed the peripheral pulse will be lost so confirming the position of the axillary artery.[26]

- A doppler probe can be useful in identifying a non-palpable axillary artery. The probe is held over the artery and a 22G needle is then inserted adjacent and parallel to the probe. Turbulence is detected by the probe if the needle is intra-arterial.[27]

- An aid to the correct placement of LA, using the Winnie perivascular technique for axillary block[28] is the feel of the site. The palpation of a "hotdog" of fluid in the axilla following injection of 40 ml LA suggests success, where as a "hamburger" indicates a subcutaneous injection and probable failure. After the arm has been returned to the side the "hotdog" can be massaged towards the axilla until it is no longer palpable.[29]

- Local anaesthesia will normally spread around the artery.

- Two needles may be needed; anterior for the ulnar nerve superficially and the median nerve deeper, posterior for the radial nerve.

- No anaesthesia to the medial upper arm. The intercostal brachial nerve has been missed. If operating above the elbow infiltrate 5–10 ml LA in a band subcutaneously just below the original injection from over the axillary artery posteriorly. The nerve lies superficial to the axillary artery.

- No anaesthesia to the lateral forearm. The musculo-cutaneous nerve has been missed. Inject 5 ml to the lateral border of biceps about 5 cm above the antecubital fossa.

Intravenous regional anaesthesia

- Venous pressures in the cubital fossa were measured distal to an inflated tourniquet as 40 ml of normal saline was injected. The rate of rise and maximum venous pressures increased with higher injection rates, failure to exsanguinate the arm and the more proximal the site of injection. For this reason the antecubital fossa should never be used for intravenous regional anaesthesia.[30]

- Interosseous vessels in children, not obstructed by a tourniquet, make this technique unsafe for children.

- The vascular volume of the forearm venous system in a 70 kg man is 17.7 ml (s.d. 4.7)[31] and it is presumed that most of this is removed by exsanguination. Therefore if a positive aspiration is made during slow IV injection it is likely that there is a leaky cuff. Aspiration has been used to detect tourniquet failure in 11 out of 128 blocks [32]

- The addition of 50 µg fentanyl and 0.5 mg pancuronium to 100 mg lidocaine diluted in 40 ml gives good analgesia and relaxation for upper limb surgery.[33]

Intra-arterial local anaesthesia

- Intra-arterial local anaesthesia has been used for a lady with severe rheumatoid arthritis and poor veins. The radial artery was cannulated, an upper arm tourniquet was inflated to 100 mmHg above systolic blood pressure; 15 ml of 0.5% lidocaine, without adrenaline, was injected over 30 s. At the start of the injection the patient experienced a burning sensation which passed rapidly. Sensation was lost within 3 min. Intra-arterial analgesia was first described in 1912.[34]

Arm blocks at the wrist

Ulnar nerve

- Identify the flexor carpi ulnaris on the ulnar side of the wrist. The palmar branch of the ulnar nerve lies lateral to flexor carpi ulnaris but medial to the ulnar artery which can usually be palpated; 2–4 ml of LA lateral to the tendon and 5 ml subcutaneously around the ulnar side of the wrist, at the level of the ulnar styloid, will block the dorsal branch and sensation to the medial one and a half fingers.

- Median nerve lies deep medial to flexor carpi radialis and lateral to palmaris longus (if present). Two ml of LA will block this nerve in its small space in the retinaculum.

- Radial nerve can be felt as its terminal branches pass over the abductor hallucis tendon at the base of the thumb. Five ml of LA, infiltrated from the palmar to the dorsal surface of the radial side of the wrist at the radial styloid process will block sensation to the dorsum of the hand

Chest

Intercostal block

There are a number of ways by which intercostal injections can be effective apart from a direct effect on the intercostal nerve. Local anaesthetic may spread to the intrapleural, paravertebral and epidural

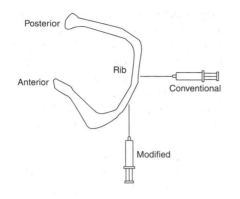

Figure 27 – Intercostal block in children: "Walk needle off parallel to rib".

spaces. A single injection of 20 ml 0.5% bupivacaine at T10 intercostal space can be as effective as 4 ml given at each of T7 to T11 for pain relief following cholecystectomy.[35,36] The intercostal space is very vascular and epinephrine should always be added to these solutions.

Intercostal blockade in children is made safer by walking a needle off the caudal edge of the rib but then angling the needle posteriorly. Advance the needle medially and posteriorly so that it is parallel to the rib and 1–2 mm below the rib. The bevel faces cephalad. A loss of resistance is detected when the needle enters the subcostal space[37] (Figure 27).

Intrapleural block

- Use. Pain relief: fractured ribs, unilateral abdominal incisions, carcinoma of pancreas and stomach.

- When used for postoperative analgesia following simple breast surgery and axillary node dissection is performed, a catheter must also be placed in the axilla. This is best sited by the surgeon, before skin closure, to give continuous brachial plexus analgesia.[38]

- Pancreatic pain is transmitted through the splanchnic nerves and parietal peritoneal pain through intercostal nerves. Both nerve pathways are affected by a left intrapleural block.[39] The intrapleural catheter can be left in place for at least 2 months.

Technique

- The patient lies on the painless side. The angle of the sixth rib is identified. The skin is infiltrated with LA over the rib and a Tuohy needle injected down to the rib and then walked off the rib until it rests under the rib but not in the pleural cavity. The needle opening is turned to face anteriorly and a catheter passed. As the catheter passes between the inner and innermost muscle layers it breaks through the innermost layer into the pleural cavity a few cm anteriorly and avoids a direct opening into the pleura.

- A number of other techniques have been suggested for avoiding a pneumothorax.

- The patient lies laterally on the painless side. A 2 ml syringe half filled with saline is connected to a three-way tap and then to a Tuohy needle. The Tuohy needle is introduced vertically over the side of the rib. When the needle enters the intrapleural space the fluid level suddenly drops. The three-way tap is closed to the patient while a catheter is threaded through the syringe and then opened to pass into the intrapleural space.[40–42] (Figure 28).

- A 16G Tuohy needle is fitted with a haemostatic valve and Luer lock intended for use with a 7G central vein. An infusion of 0.9% saline is connected to the side port of the valve and the system flushed with saline to exclude air. The line is then clamped shut. Once the Tuohy needle is

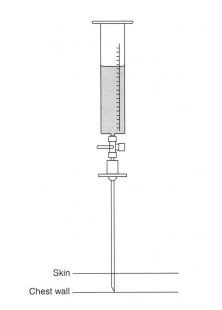

Skin ——————

Chest wall ——————

Figure 28 – Falling column to identify intrapleural space.

in the subcutaneous tissue the clamp is opened and a few drops of saline will flow into the tissues. When the subpleural space is traversed a few drops of saline will enter the drip chamber. As the parietal pleura is breached there is a free flow of saline. An extradural catheter can be passed through the flap valve into the pleural cavity. The Tuohy needle is now withdrawn and at no time can air enter the pleural cavity.[43]

- Twenty ml bupivacaine 0.25–0.5% with 1:200,000 epinephrine can give 6–8 h pain relief.

- It may be advisable to have the patient supine when administering any volume of LA into the intrapleural space in order to prevent phrenic nerve paralysis.[44,45]

Paravertebral block

- Use. Cervical region. A block of the anterior primary rami of C3 and C4 gives pain relief for carotid artery and thyroid

surgery and internal jugular cannulation. The approach is as for an interscalene brachial plexus block but higher. Identify the transverse process of C6 opposite the cricoid cartilage. Then the transverse processes of C4 and C3. A 21G needle is injected onto the lateral aspect of the processes coming from above downwards to touch the bone of the process before entering the vertebral artery. After aspirating, 2–3 ml of LA is injected. The concentration of LA should be limited to a sensory block at C4 to avoid a phrenic nerve palsy.

- Use. Upper thoracic region from C7 to T5 for breast and axillary surgery[46] and chest pain. Patient sitting or prone. Identify the spines of C7 to T5. C7 is the most prominent spine in the neck and is grooved. A line drawn laterally from the upper border of the spine overlies the transverse process. Introduce a 20–22G 10 cm needle on this line, 3.5 cm lateral to the mid-line, until it reaches the bone of the transverse process. Redirect the needle to pass below or above the process and introduce for a further 2 cm until the needle passes through the costotransverse ligament and loss of resistance to injection is detected. Aspirate and then inject 3 ml 0.5% bupivacaine with epinephrine into each space. A catheter can be passed using a Tuohy needle to one space. Note that above C7 is C7 nerve root, above T1 is C8 nerve root, below T1 is T1 root. A block with 15 ml bupivacaine at T3–4 may give relief for intractable angina. Side effects: bradycardia, pneumothorax, epidural block and Horner's syndrome.

- Use. Lower thoracic region. The point lateral to the upper border of the spine overlies the transverse process of the verteba below. The depth to the transverse process increases up to 5 cm.

- From T12 caudally the line drawn laterally from the spine overlies the caudal edge of transverse process of the same vertebra. If the needle is advanced too far it will enter psoas, but not cause a pneumothorax. The depth to the transverse process is 4–5 cm but can be more.

- At L2 or L3 the needle can be passed through the paravertebral space until resistance to injection is felt in psoas muscle. A lumber plexus block is made by injecting 20 ml of LA into psoas.

Epidural and spinal block

Position

- Sitting. Arms over a pillow flexes the spine. Ideal for upper thoracic and cervical as well as lumbar access. Patient may become hypotensive and faint. The elderly can be supported by an assistant on each side and gentle traction applied under the arms to lift the patient and open up the intervertebral spaces.

- Lateral. Easier for image intensifier.

- Mark the interspinous space by gently indenting the skin with the thumb nail (Figure 29).

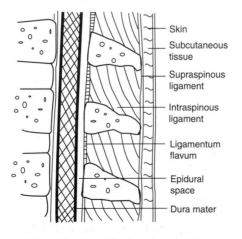

Figure 29 – Sagittal section of vertebral column.

Skin
Subcutaneous tissue
Supraspinous ligament
Intraspinous ligament
Ligamentum flavum
Epidural space
Dura mater

- Mark the mid-line with index and middle fingers in the paravertebral space.

- The obese can be a problem if no spines are felt. In the sitting position ask the patient, with their own finger, to point to the centre of their back. They will do this with remarkable accuracy so that the sagittal plain can be identified. Infiltrate skin and subcutaneous tissue with LA and use a 10 cm needle to ensure that you are injecting between two spines.[47]

Preparing the site when the patient is sitting:

- Paper drapes can fall off and get in the way. An alternative is to clean the skin with antiseptic and then a transparent adhesive dressing is applied over the site for injection. The needle is injected through the dressing. The adhesive dressing can be left in place and a second dressing applied to fix the catheter.[48]

Where is L4 in adults?

- A line drawn between the uppermost part of the iliac crests has been used as a guide to the level of L4–5. This line is known as Jacoby's line in Japan. He described the guideline in: *New York Medical Journal* 1895; **62:** 813–18. This was 5 years before Tuffier's description in *Seminars in Medicine* 1900; **20:** 167–9.[49]

- The line drawn between the highest point of the iliac crests (intercristal line) crosses the mid-line at the level of L5 vertebrae in children and at the L5–S1 interspace in neonates. This line is therefore a guide to a safe level for injection into the CSF below the spinal cord, which stops at about L1.[50]

Approach to epidural space

- The paramedian approach to the lumbar epidural space may have two advantages over the mid-line approach. In cadavers the epidural needle travels a longer distance in the epidural space from the paramedian approach reducing the risk of dural puncture. The catheter from the paramedian approach does not dent the dura and takes a straight cephalad approach.[51]

Detection of epidural space

There are several ways of detecting the epidural space. Most are based on loss of resistance as the needle passes through the ligamentum flavum or the detection of negative pressure within the space.

- The negative pressure within the space can be detected by fitting a piece of IV tubing or the clear plastic sheath, as supplied with some epidural kits, onto the hub of the Tuohy needle. The tubing is filled with a few drops of 0.9% saline, before being attached.[52,53]

- Some tissues offer little resistance to the advancing Tuohy needle. This may be a problem if the needle is exactly in the mid-line where the ligaments meet. Resistance to injection can then be tested before and after firm sideways tilting of the needle, in a direction opposite to the bevel. Tilting compresses the tissues and increases the resistance to injection. If the resistance increases on tilting the needle it can be safely advanced. Once the needle is in the epidural space tilting makes no difference to the resistance[54] (Figure 29).

- Two ml of air injected into the epidural space gives a whoosh sound heard through a stethoscope over the thoraco lumbar region. When air is injected into the subcutaneous tissue a high pitched crackling noise is heard.[55,56]

- A small amount of fluid added to the air converts the whoosh to a loud crunch.[57]

- Moore's air test for a caudal block.[58] A stethoscope is placed over the upper lumbar region, close to the mid-line; 2–5 ml of air is rapidly injected after a negative aspiration test. Correct placement of the needle is associated with a loud crunching noise, if the needle is outside the caudal canal no sound is heard.

- Sound in the Tuohy needle. A stethoscope is connected to a three-way tap placed between the Tuohy needle and a loss of resistance syringe. As the needle passes through the ligaments a cutting noise is heard. The sound increases when the ligamentum flavum is cut. This is followed by a sucking sound on entering the epidural space.[59]

- In children the epidural space can be identified using an intravenous microdrip infusion of saline. The infusion chamber is kept at about 1 m above the puncture site. When the injecting needle is in the intraspinous ligament no dripping is observed. When the needle is in the epidural space there is a free flow of fluid in the drip chamber.[60]

- Loss of resistance using a syringe containing saline plus a bulb of air gives the syringe contents a degree of compressibility for bounce and sensitivity, while saline is injected into the epidural space.[61] The air bubble acts as a spirit level to ensure that the needle is kept horizontal. If the fluid can be injected without compressing the bubble this indicates correct placement in the epidural space.[62]

- Once the epidural catheter is in place the open end is raised to the level of the uppermost iliac crest. The fluid level will fall if it is correctly in the epidural space. If the catheter is lowered the fluid level will rise.[63]

- Use a Queckenstedt test when no CSF emerges but the needle is suspected of being in the subdural space. Bilateral pressure on the jugular veins, raises the intracranial pressure by obstructing the flow of blood outwards. This in turn increases the pressure in the spinal canal and creates a free flow of CSF through the needle.[64]

The catheter passes easier and avoids puncturing blood vessels if 4–6 ml of LA is injected into the space, after a test dose of 2 ml, rather than introducing the catheter into a dry space.[65]

Pain in the epidural space

- For patient comfort only saline should be injected into the epidural space as water causes pain. The pain caused by injecting water can be used as a positive way of identifying the epidural space.[66–68]

- Pain can be used to confirm placement of LA in the epidural space. There may be a sharp pain on injection, possibly due to cold fluid. Deepening of respiration on injection may link to this stimulus. If a large volume is injected pain occurs between the shoulder blades.

- Interscapular pain during epidural topup may be due to meningeal stretching. A pain on neck flexion (L'Hermitte's phenomenon) is experienced by MS patients possibly due to a direct mechanical effect on the spinal cord.[69] When the pain is severe the rate of infusion should be reduced or stopped.

- Paraesthesia and shooting pain to the leg when the catheter is passed suggests irritation of a nerve root.[70]

- Headache occurring during or after an epidural injection in a pre-eclamptic patient may indicate the presence of cerebral oedema. This in turn is an early sign of impending eclampsia.[71]

Deafness and vertigo

- Spinal anaesthesia can lead to complete hearing loss, relieved by a blood patch. A reduced CSF pressure is linked to a low intralabyrinthine pressure which reduces the ability of the ear to transmit high tones.[72]

- An extradural injection can be associated with reversible vertigo and nausea, tinnitus and deafness. The mechanism is not clear.[73]

Spinal tap

- None of the temperature, pH, presence of glucose or turbidity tests are reliable in distinguishing between LA and CSF.[74]

- Spinal headache is often occipital but also over the crown, frontal or between the shoulder blades. It is aggravated by sitting and there may be neck stiffness.

- Pain in the orbit is a feature of a dural tap. It can occur within an hour of the tap.[75]

- Diplopia due to a sixth nerve palsy is probably due to traction on the nerve during its long intracranial course.

What to do with a dural tap?

- Insert a catheter at another level.

- Consider: Hold the Tuohy needle in the subdural space, particularly if it has been difficult to find the vertebral canal and introduce a catheter into the subarachnoid space. A volume of 2–3 ml bupivacaine 0.25% every 2–3 h will be sufficient to produce good analgesia with sensory loss. Any hypotension will be more rapid in onset and should be treated quickly with fluids and ephedrine. A lower concentration of bupivacaine will provide analgesia without profound sensory loss.[76] This is useful for managing the very sick or terminally ill patient, enabling the better titration of dose and volume against effect.

Postlumbar puncture headache

A number of studies have shown that bed rest may postpone the headache but it does not lessen the incidence nor prevent it.[77–81]

- Early mobilisation is recommended after lumbar puncture performed for diagnostic reasons or radiological procedures.

- A blood patch of up to 30 ml will halt the headache; 20–30 ml blood is taken aseptically and injected slowly to avoid shoulder pain. The patient remains supine for 30 min. Pre-treatment with an anticholinergic should be considered as a blood patch can cause a significant bradycardia at the time of injection.[82]

- ACTH 1.5 μg/kg infused over 1 h in 1 or 2 l of Ringer lactate will relieve the headache by the end of the infusion but it returns if the patient walks immediately afterwards. During the next 6–12 h final relief is established. A side effect is a reduced requirement for hypoglycaemic agents in diabetic patients.[83,84]

- Caffeine sodium benzoate 500 mg given in 1 l of intravenous crystalloid fluid and followed, if necessary, by a second 500 mg in 1 l after 4 h relieves 70% of patients with postdural puncture headache.[85]

- Carbon dioxide, inhaled intermittently, increases CSF production.

Betadine as a cause of pain

- Betadine contains a number of toxic chemicals. Small amounts of betadine can be carried into the CSF where it will cause irritation and pain. In one study betadine caused pain in 6% of patients.[86] All cleaning fluids should be either allowed to dry or wiped away before passing a needle through the area.[87]

Dimensions of the epidural space

- The mean distance from skin to the lumbar epidural space in neonates is 1 cm; older infants and children either, depth (cm) $= 1 + (0.15 \times \text{age in years})$, or depth (cm) $= 0.8 + (0.05 \times \text{weight (kg)})$[88]; adults 3–5 cm except in the obese when a 150 mm needle may be required.

- A guide to the volume (ml) of solution to block one segment is the age plus 2 divided by 10 in children.[89] In adults allow 2 ml per segment but less in the thoracic and cervical region, obstetric and the elderly patient.

- The volume of bupivacaine for use in spinal block has been recorded as 0.22 ml per spinal segment. The level of sensory block does not relate to the patients' physical status.[90]

- Caudal block in children. Perineal operations LA dose: Under 10 years old, dose $= 1$ mg/kg weight. Over 10 years old, dose $= 0.1$ ml $\times$ age in years for each dermatome to be blocked. For perineal operations 0.5 ml/year of age, for inguinal operations 1.0 ml/year of age, up to 2 mg/kg.

Securing an epidural catheter

Epidural catheters migrate both inwards and outwards. Fixation is a problem. Solutions offered include:

- Attach catheter onto two circular double stick plasters, one at the site of catheter entry to the skin and the other 5 cm away. The whole is covered by a transparent adhesive dressing.[91]

- To allow the patient to wash and particularly to shower an ostomy bag can be placed over the catheter. The catheter is first secured with steristrips to skin within a 7 cm diameter of the skin puncture. The catheter is threaded through the baseplate of the stoma bag which is secured to the skin. The catheter is coiled up to fit the ostomy bag.[92]

- A square of the adhesive gum pad, used for fixing colostomy bags to the skin, will cover the catheter and hold it to the skin.

Removing the catheter

- A trapped catheter will often be released by flexion and rotation of the spine. The patient may sit or lie on their side with the back flexed. A nurse vigorously flexes the patient into a chin knee position. The catheter is then pulled free.[93]

Care should be exercised as to the best time to remove a catheter when the patient is receiving an anticoagulant. Remove before the next dose of prophylactic heparin and never while fully anticoagulated.

Drugs for continuous infusion

Pain relief is obtained with epidural bupivacaine 0.125–0.25% plus a lipid soluble opioid added – fentanyl 50 μg. Pethidine 50 mg has analgesic and LA properties. Clonidine 50 μg is also added.

Spinal block pain relief: bupivacaine 0.0625–0.125% with fentanyl 10–25 μg or pethidine 5–10 mg and/or clonidine 10–25 μg.

Assess the level of the block

- Dermatome levels: above clavicle C4, below clavicle T2, nipple T4, xiphisternum T6, umbilicus T10, groin T12, upper thigh L1, knee L3, medial thigh L4, lateral thigh and hallux L5, fifth toe S1 (Figures 30 and 31).

- Cold from ethyl chloride spray, alcohol swab or a metal stethoscope is used for detecting the level of a block.[94]

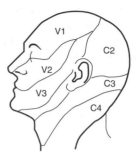

Figure 30 – Cranial dermatomes.

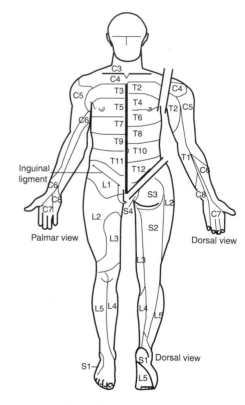

Figure 31 – Body dermatomes.

- A controlled pin prick.

- The current from a nerve stimulator can be applied to the skin starting with a low, followed by a higher amplitude, at 2, followed by 50 Hz. A sensation of paraesthesia is detected in normally innervated skin. In slender patients stimulation of the intercostal nerves leads to contraction of the muscles of the chest and abdominal wall.[95]

Identifying a dural tap

- If there is doubt that a spinal puncture has been performed, pressure applied bilaterally to the jugular veins raises intracranial pressure and creates a flow of CSF through a spinal needle.[64]

- The use of fine needles for spinal blockade means that CSF may not be readily seen. The dura can be identified better when the epidural space has been entered using a Tuohy needle and loss of resistance to saline is used. The spinal needle is now passed through the epidural needle containing saline or if air has been used a small meniscus of saline is formed in the hub of the epidural needle. When the dura is indented the meniscus is drawn in. When the dura has been punctured the meniscus returns out again and finally CSF returns up the spinal needle.[96]

Caudal block

- Use. Pain relief in perineum.

- The epidural space runs from the foramen magnum to the sacral hiatus. The lower end can be entered through the sacral hiatus.

- The patient is placed prone with feet internally rotated to relax the gluteal muscles. A right handed person stands to the left of the patient and runs their left index finger up the coccyx until a step is felt where the spine of S5 should be. A 21G needle is injected under the finger into the step at about 45° to the skin until it touches bone. The needle is redirected more horizontally into the sacral canal. Loss of resistance to injection confirms the epidural space which contains veins at this level. It is essential to aspirate before injecting 10 ml LA to block the sacral nerve roots.

Sympathetic blocks

The efferent sympathetic pathway starts in the hypothalamus and passes through the brainstem to form the lateral horn in the thoracic spinal cord. Sympathetic nerves only leave with the T1 to L1 nerve roots to synapse in the sympathetic ganglia antero-lateral to the vertebrae or pass through these ganglia to other ganglia.

Stellate ganglion

Use. Sympathetic pain in arm, head and neck, angina.

Anatomy: the stellate ganglion is formed of the inferior cervical and the first thoracic ganglion. It lies anterior to the head of the first rib and antero-lateral to the body of T1 and C7, in the prevertebral fascia.

- A safe and specific technique uses an image intensifier to identify the body of C7. A 100 mm, 22G needle is introduced lateral to the trachea and medial to the carotid artery onto the anterior lateral body of C7 and withdrawn 5 mm off the periosteum. One ml of Niopam 200 will confirm the position. Local anaesthetic of 5–10 ml is injected.

- A blind approach must avoid the pleura and is made at the level of the cricoid cartilage C6 with the patient 45° head up. The needle enters two fingers above and two fingers lateral to the sternal notch or directly over the transverse process of C6. The fingers draw the carotid sheath laterally and the needle is injected between the retracting fingers and the trachea. Once the bone is felt, withdraw the needle 5 mm out of the fascia and inject 5–10 ml LA.

- A block will give Horner's syndrome of, unilateral ptosis, miosis, enophthalmos, anhydrosis, dilatation of the vessels of arm and face and nasal stuffiness.

Coeliac plexus block

- Use. Recommend for cancer pain of the upper abdominal viscera and of the pelvic organs. Chronic pain such as pancreatitis tends to return after a variable time, usually months.

- Anatomy: the plexus lies around the coeliac artery anterior to the body of L1.

- Precautions: this block will affect all sympathetic nerves below the diaphragm. The patient should be preloaded with 1–2 l of crystalloid and the blood pressure monitored. Ephedrine may be required. The patient lies prone with pillows supporting the chest and legs.

- A blind technique for coeliac plexus block, described by Moore,[97] uses a point of entry for the needle no more than 7 cm lateral to the mid-line at about L1, below the costal margin. The needle tip is passed until it lies 1.5 cm antero-lateral to the vertebral body of L1.

- L1 is located using an image intensifier with a lateral view. The coeliac plexus is clustered anteriorly to L1 around the coeliac artery. To pass a needle from the skin to the plexus the needle must go lateral to the transverse processes of the lumbar vertebrae and through the diaphragmatic crura. In practice the needles are inserted at about the level of L2, as far lateral as the ribs will allow, and passed cephalad and medial to the renal parenchyma. The needles aim to touch the waste of the vertebral body at L1. Pressure on the periosteum is painful so no force is used, but the needle is withdrawn slightly and redirected to lie antero-lateral to the

body. The inferior vena cava is on the right and aorta is on the left. Aspirate and inject 0.5 ml of a contrast fluid which will spread in the prevertebral space to the vertebra above and below. The depth of needle penetration is 11–15 cm.

Injection

- First 2 ml of LA is injected as the patient will experience a severe kick in the stomach due to alcohol. Moore recommends 25 ml of absolute alcohol through each needle. Another technique uses a mixture of 25 ml absolute alcohol with 18 ml 0.75% bupivacaine and 7 ml radio opaque contrast medium.[98]

- Fifty ml of 50% alcohol anteriorly to L1 gives relief of pain in 85% of patients with no long-term side effects. A large volume allows greater latitude in needle placement than small volumes[99] but volumes of 10 ml on each side are effective. When tumour is present it is advisable to try to inject on both sides and give a larger volume as the tumour can prevent spread of the solution.

Lumbar sympathetic chain

- Use. Pain due to leg ischaemia, cancer of pelvis.

- Anatomy: The lumbar sympathetic chain lies antero-lateral to the bodies of lumbar 2, 3 and 4 vertebrae and anterior to psoas and iliacus. The patient lies prone for a bilateral injection or in a lateral position for an unilateral injection. Blind injection is not recommended as it is impossible to be certain of the level and to avoid an intervertebral arch injection. If no X-ray is available the needle is introduced 2–3 cm lateral to the cephalad end of the spine of each vertebra, corresponding to the ganglia to be blocked. L2 affects the thigh, L3 the calf and L4 the foot. The transverse process lies deep to this point. Once the needle has touched the transverse process the needle is walked off caudally and advanced by 3 cm to the anterior lateral vertebral body.

- Aspirate.

- Injection should be without resistance: 5 ml of 6% aqueous phenol at each sympathetic ganglion or 15 ml at L3 to spread to L2 and L4. Advise the patient to drink copiously for 24 h to prevent an effect of the phenol on the kidney.

The use of the image intensifier is preferred because it

- allows accurate location of each vertebral level and site of injection,

- allows a more lateral approach (5 cm from the mid-line) to avoid touching transverse process, periosteum and nerve roots,

- confirms the placement by 0.5 ml X-ray contrast fluid, anterior to the vertebral bodies and away from epidural and dural spaces or intravascular injection.

Abdomen

Rectus sheath

- Use. Pain relief for laparoscopy and umbilical hernia repair in children.

- A four-point injection, either side of the mid-line, with up to 30 ml bupivacaine (maximum 2 mg/kg/4 h) plus epinephrine.[100]

Inguinal field

- Use. Postoperative pain relief for inguinal incisions or operation in exceptional circumstances.

- Two considerations with inguinal field block are the use of large volumes of LA, thus the addition of epinephrine is essential, and additional infiltration

required at the internal ring to block the genitofemoral nerve and inguinal sac.

- A short bevel needle makes it easier to place the needle and LA in the correct tissue planes.

- A skin wheal of LA is raised at a point 2 cm along a line from the anterior superior iliac spine to the umbilicus. A small opening is made in the skin so that there is no skin resistance to a 22G short bevel needle. The needle is advanced for about 1 cm until a pop is felt as it penetrates the external oblique aponeurosis. Seven ml of LA is injected after a negative aspiration. The needle is advanced with pressure on the syringe through the internal oblique muscle for about 5 mm until a less distinct second pop is felt. Resistance is lost to injection at this point and 8 ml of LA is injected (Figure 32).

- Next the internal ring is located 1 cm superior to the midinguinal point. At this point the external iliac artery can be palpated and the genitofemoral nerve and indirect hernia sac are deep to the internal oblique muscle. A skin wheal of LA is made and a second skin opening made. A short bevel needle is advanced until a distinct pop is felt as the needle passes through the external oblique aponeurosis. The needle is advance until a second pop is felt with loss of resistance to injection at

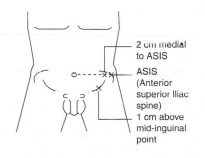

2 cm medial to ASIS

ASIS (Anterior superior iliac spine)

1 cm above mid-inguinal point

Figure 32 – Inguinal field block.

about 4 cm deep. Ten ml of LA is injected slowly.

- Thirdly the skin is infiltrated along the line of the incision with 10 ml of LA. At the lateral end of the incision line 3 ml of LA is injected subcutaneously in the line of the umbilicus. At no point is an attempt made to fan the injection of LA as it spreads in the tissues.[101]

Penile block

- Use. Penile block using 1 ml per 3 years of age of LA avoids the motor blockade of a caudal block for post-circumcision pain.

- The value of using a single mid-line needle is disputed as there is rarely free communication across the mid-line.[102] Most of the sensory innervation to the penis is in the two dorsal nerves which are terminal branches of the pudendal nerve. There is a triangular space deep to the fascia bounded above by the symphysis pubis and below by the corpora cavernosa. The fascia splits on its under side to form a vertical suspensory ligament which divides to encircle the shaft of the penis. The safest place to inject an adequate volume is deep to the fascia, on each side of the suspensory ligament. This avoids the mid-line where dorsal vessels lie deep to the ligament.

- The patient/child is supine. A short bevel needle is inserted into the two compartments of the subpubic space, where the nerves run before entering the base of the penis. The two sites for needle puncture are 0.5 (in infants) to 1 (in older children) cm lateral to the symphysis pubis and immediately below the right and left inferior rami of the pubic bone. The base of the penis is pulled down and the needle is advanced posteriorly at 70–80° angle to the skin, slightly medially and caudally. After a first "give" is felt passing through the superficial fascia, the needle is

advanced until a second "give" is felt passing through Scarp's fascia. The needle is now in the subpubic space. Local anaesthetic of 0.1 ml/kg is injected into each side.[103,104]

Superior hypogastric plexus block for pelvic pain

- The sympathetic nerves, from the pelvis, lie anterior to the pelvic promontory. With the patient prone, skin wheals are raised 5–7 cm lateral to the L4–L5 interspinous space on each side. On each side, a 22G, 7 in. needle is inserted and directed towards the mid-line, 30° caudad and 45° mesiad so that the tip lies in the retroperitoneal space antero-lateral to L5. The position of each needle is confirmed by X-ray. It may pass through the fascia of psoas with a loss of resistance. A test block using 6–8 ml 0.25% bupivacaine or a lytic block using 6–8 ml 10% aqueous phenol are used on each side[105] (Figure 33).

- Bupivacaine infiltrated into the mesosalpinx reduces the pain after ring sterilisation.[106]

Lower limb blocks

3-in-1 block

A distal approach to the femoral plexus.

- Use. Postoperative hip surgery pain (Figure 34).

- Winnie described a 3-in-1 block of obturator, femoral and lateral femoral cutaneous nerves with a single injection filling the anatomical plane between quadratus lumborum and psoas major.[107]

- The femoral nerve is located below the mid-point of the inguinal ligament, lateral to the femoral artery.

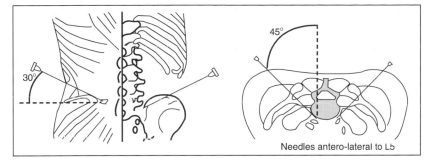

Figure 33 – Hypogastric plexus block.

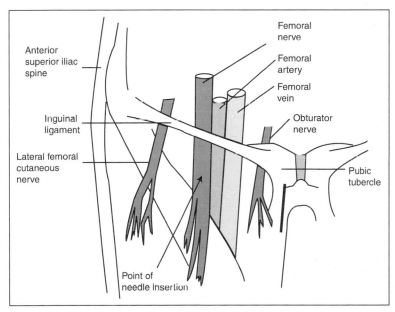

Figure 34 3-in-1 block.

- A 22G needle, or Tuohy needle if using a catheter, attached to a nerve stimulator is introduced 2–3 cm below the inguinal ligament over the position of the nerve and advanced towards the ligament at 45° to the skin. It will be felt to enter the femoral sheath and paraesthesia elicited or a contraction seen in quadratus femoris. Bupivacaine 0.25%, 20–30 ml is injected and a catheter passed and taped in place for further injections of 20 ml at intervals of 4–6 h.

A 3-in-1 block may miss the lateral cutaneous nerve of thigh. This is blocked by local anaesthetic injected deep to the fascia lata infero-medially to the anterior superior iliac spine.

A lateral cutaneous nerve of thigh block can result in a 3-in-1 block with loss of sensation in L2/3 and leg weakness. This should be borne in mind when using local anaesthetic injections for postoperative pain relief of lower abdominal incisions.[108]

Sciatic nerve block

Posterior approach

- The patient lies with the side to be blocked upper most. An assistant holds this upper leg with the knee flexed and hip flexed as far as possible with slight abduction. In this position the sciatic nerve is stretched in the hollow between the greater trochanter and the ischial tuberosity. The gluteus maximus muscle is also thinned making the nerve more superficial. The mid-point of the line between the greater trochanter and the ischial tuberosity is located. A 22G 100 mm spinal needle, attached to a nerve stimulator, is inserted perpendicularly to the skin until the best foot plantar flexion or dorsiflexion is obtained. Local anaesthetic of 20 ml is injected[109] (Figure 35).

A distal approach to the sciatic nerve, similar in principle to a 3-in-1 block, is an approach from the popliteal fossa.

- The patient is prone. With the hip flexed to 90° and the knee extended the tibial nerve can usually be located or palpated in the lateral half of the popliteal fossa, medial to biceps femoris. The common peroneal (lateral popliteal) nerve is usually palpable at the neck of the fibula and can then be traced higher as it runs parallel, deep and slightly medial to biceps femoris tendon. The position for LA at the fibula head, or in the popliteal fossa is confirmed using a nerve stimulator. A stimulation of 1.0 mA is used for the tibial nerve and 0.5 mA for the common peroneal nerve (Figure 36).

- The angle formed by biceps femoris laterally and semitendenosus medially is drawn. The angle is bisected and the lateral half of the angle is further bisected. The tibial nerve and common peroneal nerve lie below the second line. A needle introduced at 45° to the skin towards the apex of the triangle, with nerve stimulator attached, will detect the nerve sheath. A single injection of 20–30 ml bupivacaine is made, followed by a catheter for topups. Larger volumes of local anaesthetic will spread back along the nerve towards the sacral plexus.

Ankle block

Use: operations on, and pain relief of, the foot.

Saphenous nerve

- The saphenous nerve, supplies the medial calf (L4). It is blocked anterior to the medial malleolus using 4 ml at the ankle or 12 ml to the femoral nerve.[110]

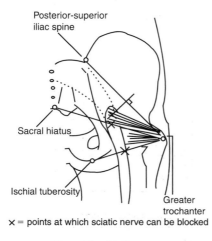

Posterior-superior iliac spine

Sacral hiatus

Ischial tuberosity

Greater trochanter

✗ = points at which sciatic nerve can be blocked

Figure 35 – Sciatic nerves.

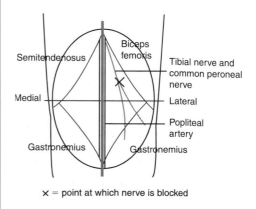

Semitendenosus

Biceps femoris

Tibial nerve and common peroneal nerve

Medial

Lateral

Popliteal artery

Gastronemius

Gastronemius

✗ = point at which nerve is blocked

Figure 36 – Sciatic nerve from popliteal fossa.

Posterior tibial nerve

- Posterior tibial nerve lies posterior to the medial malleolus. It supplies the sole of the foot except the most proximal and lateral parts. A reliable block uses a subcalcaneal approach. The point of needle insertion is defined in relationship to the sustentaculum tali, a bony prominence which is palpable 2–3 cm below the medial malleolus. The nerve passes beneath this bony landmark[111] where 2–3 ml of LA will produce a block, after aspiration to avoid the tibial artery. The nerve can be stimulated at this point to produce toe plantar flexion to assess the return of neuromuscular function.

Sural nerve

- The sural nerve lies posterior to the lateral malleolus. It is sensory to the posterior calf and a small band of skin on the medial foot. It is blocked by infiltrating 5 ml between the lateral malleolus and the Achilles tendon.

Anterior ankle nerves

- The superficial peroneal nerve lies anterior to the lateral malleolus. It supplies the dorsum of the foot and toes. LA of 5–10 ml is injected subcutaneously from the lateral malleolus to the anterior border of the tibia.

- Mid-way between the malleoli on the anterior surface of the ankle is the deep peroneal nerve which supplies the first web space; 5–10 ml LA is injected between the tendons of tibialis anterior and extensor hallucis longus, deep to the extensor retinaculum.

Lung Function

- Continuous monitoring of pressure–volume (PV) or flow–volume (QV)

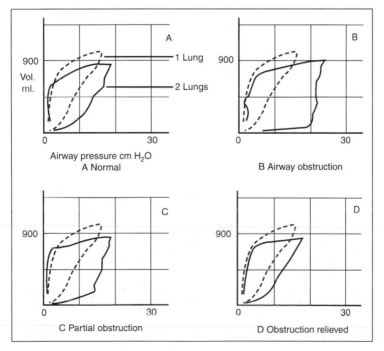

Figure 37 – Pressure–volume loops.

loops gives information about changes in airway pressure, lung compliance and airway resistance.

- The normal PV loop is illustrated in Figure 37.

The shape of the PV loop becomes more open, square or rectangular with:

- reduced compliance such as in obesity, pneumo–abdomen, the pressure of an intra–abdominal retractor;

- malposition of a tracheal tube;

- reduced airway calibre and increasing airway resistance give a bowing of the QV loop.[112]

The QV loop (Figure 38)

- A normal loop (Figure 38A) seen during anaesthesia. Inspiration starts at the point that expiration ends and reaches a steady state of flow. Expiratory flow is initially rapid in the opposite direction and returns to the original lung volume.

- Failure to complete the loop suggests air trapping within the lung as occurs in severe asthma.

- Smooth waves on the expiratory curve suggests the return of spontaneous breathing during paralysis.

- A saw tooth pattern on a QV loop during anaesthesia (Figure 38B) strongly suggests the presence of airway secretions even in the absence of clinical signs.[113]

- A leak around a cuff can be detected as a difference between inspiratory and expiratory volumes.[114]

- The flow volume loop can be used to assess lung function. A loop recorded from maximum expiration to maximum inspiration shows residual volume, and total lung capacity, peak inspiratory and peak expiratory flow rates (Figure 38C).

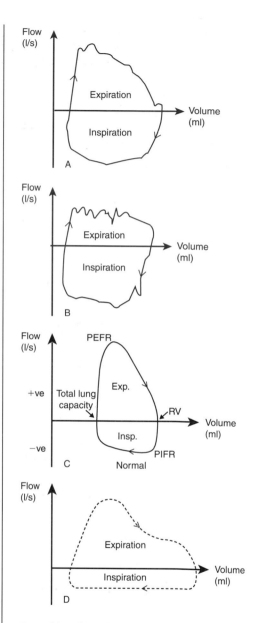

Figure 38 – Flow volume loop showing: (A) normal, (B) partially obstructed with secretions, (C) maximum expiration to maximum inspiration, (D) inspiratory obstruction, expiratory obstruction.

Obstruction to inspiration gives a flatter more prolonged inspiratory curve. Expiratory obstruction gives a lower peak followed by a dip and trough (Figure 38D).

- The QV loop can be used as a vitalograph. The patient breaths maximally out, then takes a maximum breath in, followed by a maximum breath out. The inspiratory flow is the peak inspiratory flow rate, the expiratory flow rate (PEER). The starting point is the functional residual volume and the end of inspiration is the vital capacity.

- Obstruction to inspiration flattens the inspiratory flow line as flow rate is reduced.

- Expiratory obstruction causes a lower PEFR followed by a prolonged expiration.

References

1. Spotoft H, Christensen P. Laryngeal oedema accompanying weight gain in pregnancy. *Anaesthesia* 1981; **36:** 71.
2. Dakin MJ, Yentis SM. Latex allergy: a strategy for management. *Anaesthesia* 1998; **53:** 774–81.
3. Rice ASC. Peripheral nerve damage and regional anaesthesia. *British Journal of Anaesthesia* 1995; **75:** 116.
4. De Andres JA. The blood lancet in regional anaesthesia. *British Journal of Anaesthesia* 1989; **62:** 348.
5. Santos DJ, Juneja M, Bridenbaugh PO. A device for uniform testing of sensory neural blockade during regional anesthesia. *Anesthesia and Analgesia* 1987; **66:** 581–2.
6. Miranda DR. Identification of the brachial plexus perivascular space. *Anaesthesia* 1977; **49:** 721–2.
7. Hamilton RC. Techniques of orbital regional anaesthesia. *British Journal of Anaesthesia* 1995; **75:** 88–92.
8. Fry RA, Henderson J. Local anaesthesia for eye surgery. *Anaesthesia* 1990; **45:** 14–17.
9. Hamilton RC. Techniques of orbital regional anaesthesia. *British Journal of Anaesthesia* 1995; **75:** 88–92.
10. Brahma AK, Pemberton CJ, Ayeko M, Morgan LH. Single medial injection peribulbar anaesthesia using prilocaine. *Anaesthesia* 1994; **49:** 1003–105.
11. Xifaras GP. Single medial injection peribulbar anaesthesia. *British Journal of Anaesthesia* 1995; **75:** 668.
12. Henthorn RW, Amayem A, Ganta R. Which method for intraoral glossopharyngeal nerve block is better? *Anesthesia and Analgesia* 1995; **81:** 1113–14.
13. Ramamurthy S et al. Long thoracic nerve block. *Anesthesia and Analgesia* 1990; **71:** 197–9.
14. Brull SJ. Superficial cervical plexus block for pulmonary artery catheter insertion. *Critical Care Medicine* 1992; **20:** 1362–3.
15. Wassef MR. Suprascapular nerve block. *Anaesthesia* 1992; **47:** 120–4.
16. Meyer-Witting M, Foster JMG. Suprascapular nerve block in the management of cancer pain. *Anaesthesia* 1992; **47:** 626.
17. Ristall JE, Sharwood-Smith GH. Suprascapular nerve block. New indications and a safer technique. *Anaesthesia* 1992; **47:** 626.
18. Parris WCV. Suprascapular nerve block: a safer technique. *Anesthesiology* 1990; **72:** 580–1.
19. Ganta R, Cajee RA, Henthorn RW. Use of transcutaneous nerve stimulation to assist interscalene block. *Anesthesia and Analgesia* 1993; **76:** 914.
20. Brown AR, Broccolli E. An aid to the performance of interscalene blocks. *Anesthesiology* 1992; **76:** 869–70.
21. Wiener DN, Speer KP. The deltoid sign. *Anesthesia and Analgesia* 1994; **79:** 192.
22. Smith BE. Distribution of evoked paraesthesia and effectiveness of brachial plexus block. *Anaesthesia* 1986; **41:** 1112–15.
23. Hickey R, Garland TA, Ramamurthy S. Subclavian perivascular block: influence of location of paraesthesia. *Anesthesia and Analgesia* 1989; **68:** 767–71.
24. Hill DA, Campbell WI. Two approaches to the axillary brachial plexus. *Anaesthesia* 1992; **47:** 207–9.
25. Yee KF. Tourniquet technique for axillary block. *Anaesthesia* 1996; **51:** 1186.
26. de Jong RH, Thurman BH. Localising the axillary artery. *Anesthesia and Analgesia* 1983; **62:** 701.
27. Abramowitz HB, Cohen C. Use of doppler for difficult axillary block. *Anesthesiology* 1981; **55:** 603.
28. Winnie AP, Collins VJ. The subclavian perivascular technique of brachial plexus anaesthesia. *Anesthesiology* 1964; **25:** 353–63.
29. Shutt L. Axillary brachial plexus block: choice of technique? *British Journal of Anaesthesia* 1990; **65:** 438.
30. El-Hassan KM, Hutton P, Black AMS. Venous pressure and arm volume changes

during simulated Bier's block. *Anaesthesia* 1984; **39:** 229–35.

31. Ploudre G, Barry PP, Tardif L, Hardy JF. Decreasing the toxic potential of intravenous regional anaesthesia. *Canadian Journal of Anaesthesia* 1989; **36:** 498–502.

32. Gurmarnik S. A simple aspiration test can detect tourniquet failure during i.v. regional anaesthesia. *British Journal of Anaesthesia* 1993; **71:** 462–3.

33. Abdulla WY, Fadhil NM. A new approach to intravenous regional anesthesia. *Anesthesia and Analgesia* 1992; **75:** 597–601.

34. Koscielniak-Nielsen ZJ, Stens-Pedersen HL. Intra-arterial regional analgesia of the hand. *British Journal of Anaesthesia* 1991; **66:** 719–20.

35. Kirno K, Lindell K. Intercostal nerve blockade. *British Journal of Anaesthesia* 1986; **58:** 246.

36. Crossley AWA, Hosie HE. Radiological study of intercostal nerve blockade in healthy volunteers. *British Journal of Anaesthesia* 1987; **59:** 149–54.

37. Shelly MP, Park GR. Intercostal nerve blockade for children. *Anaesthesia* 1987; **42:** 541–4.

38. Velasco RJ et al. Combined interpleural analgesia/continuous brachial plexus block for breast surgery; a new solution for a problem? *Anesthesia and Analgesia* 1993; **77:** 1077.

39. Durrani Z, Winnie AP, Ikuta P. Interpleural catheter analgesia for pancreatic pain. *Anesthesia and Analgesia* 1988; **67:** 479–81.

40. Ben-David B. The falling column: a new technique for interpleural catheter placement. *Anaesthesia and Analgesia* 1990; **71:** 212.

41. Lee E, Ben-David B. Identification of the interpleural space. *British Journal of Anaesthesia* 1990; **65:** 130.

42. Marsh B, McDonald P. A modified technique for the insertion of an interpleural catheter. *Anaesthesia* 1991; **46:** 889.

43. Scott PV. Interpleural regional analgesia: detection of the interpleural space by saline infusion. *British Journal of Anaesthesia* 1991; **66:** 131–3.

44. Gallart L et al. Intrapleural analgesia, phrenic nerve paralysis and patient position. *Anaesthesia* 1994; **49:** 175.

45. Lauder GR. Interpleural analgesia and phrenic nerve palsy. *Anaesthesia* 1993; **48:** 315–16.

46. Coveney E, Weltz CR, Greengrass R et al. Use of paravertebral block anesthesia in the surgical management of breast cancer. *Annals of Surgery* 1998; **227:** 496–501.

47. Bird J. An aid to epidural or subarachnoid location. *Anaesthesia* 1994; **49:** 923.

48. Ellermeyer WP. A modification of traditional sterile technique for regional anesthesia. *Anesthesiology* 1987; **67:** 150–1.

49. Kubota Y, Toyoda Y, Kubota H. Jacoby's line rather than Tuffier's line as a guide to lumbar puncture. *Anesthesia and Analgesia* 1992; **74:** 939.

50. Busoni P, Messeri A. Spinal anesthesia in children: surface anatomy. *Anesthesia and Analgesia* 1989; **68:** 418–19.

51. Blomberg RG. Technical advantages of the paramedian approach for lumbar epidural puncture and catheter introduction. *Anaesthesia* 1988; **43:** 837–43.

52. Tillman HA, Bhatia KN. Another, yet simpler device for the identification of the epidural space. *Anesthesiology* 1984; **60:** 79–80.

53. Mustafa K, Milliken RA. A simple, device for identification of the epidural space. *Anesthesiology* 1982; **57:** 330–2.

54. Brandstater B. The needle tilt test: an aid to epidural needle insertion. *Anesthesiology* 1989; **70:** 366–7.

55. Lewis MPN, Thomas P, Wilson LF, Mullholland RC. The "whoosh" test. *Anaesthesia* 1992; **47:** 57–8.

56. Mantha S. Origin of the "Whoosh" test. *Anaesthesia* 1993; **47:** 94

57. Lee ME, Whoosh test. *Anaesthesia* 1992; **47:** 451–2.

58. Moore DC. Regional Block, 4th edn. Thomas, Chicago 1981; p 447; referred to in: Lee ME. Identification of the caudal epidural space. *Anaesthesia* 1988; **43:** 705–6.

59. Jacob S, Tierney E. A dual technique for identification of the epidural space. *Anaesthesia* 1997; **52:** 141–3.

60. Yamashita M, Tsuji M. Identification of the epidural space in children. *Anaesthesia* 1991; **46:** 872–4.

61. Wait CM. Identification of the epidural space. *Anaesthesia* 1987; **42:** 1231.

62. Dornan RV. A useful method of identifying the epidural and caudal space. *Anaesthesia* 1994; **49:** 556.

63. Daykin AP. A test to show correct placement of epidural catheter. *Anaesthesia* 1982; **37:** 863.

64. Dvir E. Queckenstedt's test in spinal anaesthesia. *Anaesthesia* 1985; **40:** 1018.

65. Verniquet AJW. Vessel puncture with epidural catheters. *Anaesthesia* 1980; **35:** 660–2.

66. Miguel R, Morse S, Reed Murtagh F. Epidural air associated with multiradicular syndrome. *Anesthesia and Analgesia* 1991; **73:** 92–4.

67. Cohen AI, Levesque PR. Saline versus water for epidural injection. *Anesthesia and Analgesia* 1993; **76:** 455–6.

68. Mayhew JF. Saline versus water for epidural injection. *Anaesthesia and Analgesia* 1993; **77:** 646.

69. Moore JK. Unexplained pain during epidural anaesthesia. *Anaesthesia* 1984; **39:** 718–19.

70. Buscher EE, Chedel D. Pain upon injection in the epidural space: common and unexplained. *Anesthesia and Analgesia* 1992; **74:** 475–6.

71. Murphy BVS, Fogarty DJ, Fitzpatrick K, Brady MM. Headache during epidural top-ups in labour – a sign of reduced intracranial compliance. *Anaesthesia and Intensive Care* 1995; **23:** 744–6.

72. Lee CM, Peachman FA. Unilateral hearing loss after spinal anaesthesia treated with epidural blood patch. *Anesthesia and Analgesia* 1986; **65:** 312–13.

73. Gordon AG, Hardy PA. Blocked ear after extradural injection. *British Journal of Anaesthesia* 1987; **59:** 666–7.

74. Tesslet MJ, Weisel S, Wahba RM, Dance DR. A comparison of simple identification tests to distinguish cerebrospinal fluid from local anaesthetic solution. *Anaesthesia* 1994; **49:** 821–2.

75. Kumar CM, Dennison B. Pain in the orbit: a feature of dural tap. *Anaesthesia* 1986; **41:** 556.

76. Morton CPJ, Swann DG. The management of accidental dural puncture in labour. *Anaesthesia* 1992; **47:** 78–9.

77. Boer WA. Bed rest after lumbar puncture is obsolete. *Anaesthesia* 1989; **444:** 934.

78. Carbatt PAT, van Crevel H. Lumbar puncture headache: controlled study on the prevention effect of 24 hours' bed rest. *Lancet* 1981; **II:** 1133–5.

79. Kauken S, Kauken L, Kannisto K, Kataja M. The prevention of headache following spinal anaesthesia. *Annales Chirurgiae et Gynaecologiae* 1981; **70:** 107–11.

80. Anderson APD, Wanscher MCJ, Huttel MS. Postspinaler kopfschmerz ist die stundige flache bettruhe eine prophylaxe? *Regional Anaesthesia* 1986; **9:** 15–17.

81. Thornberry EA, Thomas TA. Posture and post-spinal headache. A controlled trial on 80 obstetric patients. *British Journal of Anaesthesia* 1988; **60:** 195–7.

82. Ackerman WE et al. Epidural blood patch does cause a decrease in heart rate. *Anesthesia and Analgesia* 1992; **74:** 619.

83. Foster P. ACTH treatment for post-lumbar puncture headache. *British Journal of Anaesthesia* 1995; **75:** 429.

84. Collier BB. Treatment for post dural puncture headache. *British Journal of Anaesthesia* 1994; **72:** 366–7.

85. Jarvis AP, Greenawalt JW, Fagraeus L. Intravenous caffeine for postdural puncture headache. *Anesthesia and Analgesia* 1986; **65:** 316–17.

86. Gurmarnik S. Skin preparation and spinal headache. *Anaesthesia* 1988; **43:** 1057.

87. Widesmith JAW. Skin preparation and spinal headache. *Anaesthesia* 1989; **44:** 528.

88. Hasan MA, Howard RF, Lloyd-Davies AR. Depth of epidural space in children. *Anaesthesia* 1994; **49:** 1085–7.

89. Hain WR. Anaesthetic doses for extradural anaesthesia in children. *Anaesthesia* 1978; **50:** 303.

90. Farrar MD, Nolte H. Spinal analgesia using bupivacaine 0.5%. *Anaesthesia* 1982; **37:** 91.

91. Harrington BE, Kopacz DJ. Securing epidural catheters: a further modification. *Anaesthesia and Analgesia* 1990; **71:** 443.

92. Hoffman J, Rogers JN. A new dressing technique for temporary percutaneous catheters used for pain management. *Anesthesia* 1992; **76:** 482–3.

93. Sia-Kho E. How to dislodge a severely trapped epidural catheter. *Anesthesia and Analgesia.* 1992; **74:** 933.

94. Hynson JM. Another use for a precordial stethoscope. *Anesthesia and Analgesia* 1992; **74:** 931.

95. Meyer RM, McCune WJ. Assessing the level of spinal anaesthesia using a neuromuscular stimulator. *Anesthesiology* 1987; **67:** 125–7.

96. Kopacz DJ, Bainton BG. Combined spinal epidural anaesthesia. a new hanging drop. *Anesthesia and Analgesia* 1996; **82:** 433.

97. Moore DC. Regional Block; *A Handbook for Use in the Clinical Practice of Medicine and*

Surgery, 3rd edn. Springfield, Illinois, CC Thomas 1969; pp 121–37.

98. Singler RC. An improved technique for alcoholic neurolysis of the celiac plexus. *Anesthesiology* 1982; **56:** 137–41.

99. Brown DL, Bulley CK, Quiel EL. Neurolytic celiac plexus block for pancreatic cancer pain. *Anesthesia and Analgesia* 1987; **66:** 869–73.

100. Muir J, Ferguson S. The rectus sheath block – well worth remembering. *Anaesthesia* 1996; **51:** 893.

101. Sparks CJ, Rudkin GE, Agiomea K, Fa'arondo JR. Inguinal field block for adult inguinal hernia repair using a short bevel needle. *Anaesthesia and Intensive Care* 1995; **23:** 143–8.

102. Brown TCK. The anatomy related to penile block. *Anaesthesia and Intensive Care* 1993; **21:** 235–6.

103. AnaeYeoman PM, Cooke R, Hain WR. Penile block for circumcision. *Anaesthesia* 1983; **38:** 862–6.

104. Dalens B, Vanneuville G, Dechelotte P. Penile block via the subpubic space in 100 children. *Anesthesia and Analgesia* 1989; **69:** 41–5.

105. Plancarte R, Amescua C, Patt RB, Aldrete JA. Superior hypogastric plexus block for pelvic cancer pain. *British Journal of Anaesthesia* 1990: **73:** 236–9.

106. Alexander JI, Hull MGR. Rectus sheath and mesosalpinx block for laproscopic sterilisation. *Anaesthesia* 1992; **47:** 271.

107. Winnie AP, Ramamorthy S, Durrani Z. The inguinal paravascular technique of lumbar plexus anesthesia: the 3-in-1 block. *Anesthesia and Analgesia* 1973; **52:** 989–96.

108. Lonsdale M. 3-in-1 block; confirmation of Winnie's anatomical hypothesis. *Anesthesia and Analgesia* 1988; **67:** 601–2.

109. Raj PP, Parks RI, Watson TD, Jenkins MT. A new single position supine approach to sciatic femoral nerve block. *Anesthesia and Analgesia* 1975; **54:** 489–94.

110. Sparks CJ, Higeleo. Foot surgery in Vanuatu: results of combined tibial, common peroneal and saphenous nerve blocks in fifty-six patients. *Anaesthesia and Intensive Care* 1989; **17:** 336–9.

111. Wassef MR. Posterior tibial nerve block. *Anaesthesia* 1991; **46:** 841–4.

112. Bardoczky GI, Engelman E, D'Hollander A. Continuous spirometry: an aid to monitoring ventilation during operation. *British Journal of Anaesthesia* 1993; **71:** 747–51.

113. Leclerc F et al. Use of the flow-volume loop to detect secretions in ventilated children. *Intensive Care Medicine* 1996; **22:** 88.

114. Simon BA et al. An aid in the diagnosis of malpositioned double-lumen tubes. *Anesthesiology* 1992; **76:** 862.

Malignant Hyperpyrexia[1]

> Diagnosis
> Reduced arterial oxygen saturation on
>   pulse oximeter
> Increased expired carbon dioxide
> Low expired oxygen concentration
> Increasing body temperature
> Treatment
> Stop causative agents
> Hundred per cent oxygen and
>   hyperventilate
> Dantrolene 2.5 mg/kg

The diagnosis of malignant hyperpyrexia (MH) may not be obvious at first.

Consider other diagnoses: thyroid crisis, salicylate toxicity, myopathy, and recreational drugs – ecstasy, neuroleptic malignant syndrome with pyrexia, muscle rigidity and rhabdomyolysis due to antidopaminergic effects of major tranquillisers 24–72 h after their administration.

MH can present immediately, from 10 min after the administration of a causative agent but also after the end of surgery.

Causes: Volatile anaesthetic agents and suxamethonium are the most potent causes.

Signs

Some or all of the following signs may be present. Monitor carbon dioxide and oxygen in breathing circuit and temperature.

- Muscles rigidity (more than just trismus). Following suxamethonium (with or without fasciculation) or during the course of anaesthesia.

- Rapid rise in body temperature more than 1°C/h.

- Unexplained tachycardia – onset may be sudden.

- Tachypnoea, increased end-tidal carbon dioxide concentration.

- Cardiac arrhythmias.

- Unstable blood pressure.

- Low oxygen saturation, unexplained cyanosis.

- Reduced O_2 concentrate in circle breathing circuit, widening gap between inspired and expired oxygen concentrations.

- Bleeding due to disseminated intravascular coagulation.

- Blood gas analysis – reduced PaO_2, increased $PaCO_2$, reduced pH, reduced (HCO_3^-), increased (K^+).

Treatment

- Either abandon procedure or terminate surgery as soon as possible.

- Avoid or stop inhalation agents and other triggers.

- Give 100% oxygen and prevent rebreathing.

- Allow patient to hyperventilate spontaneously to clear carbon dioxide if not paralysed.

- Or hyperventilate with minute volume of 30–40 l.

- Non-depolarising muscle relaxant may be used to facilitate ventilation but may not overcome muscle spasm.

- Dantrolene by rapid IV infusion – 1 mg/kg.

- Repeat dantrolene as necessary to a total of 10 mg/kg (average requirement 2.5 mg/kg). This takes time to mix and administer.

- Give large dose of glucocorticoid e.g. methylprednisolone 2 g to the average adult.

M

- Establish monitoring: ECG rate and rhythm, BP, temperature probe – tympanic membrane. Oesophageal temperature may be lowered by influx of cold IV fluids.

  Peripheral large bore IV line for fluids and electrolytes, full blood count, clotting screen.

  Arterial cannulation for blood gas, potassium, creatinine kinase and BP.

  Central venous cannulation for fluid balance.

- When possible

  Urinary catheter, urine output, myoglobinuria.

  Fluid output and fluid balance. Fluid loss from sweating may be high.

- Cooling and rehydration:

  Cold IV fluids: 0.9% saline (at least 1–2 1 initially) not Hartman's solution (contains potassium).

  Use blood warmer filled with iced water to cool IV fluids.

  Surface cooling with ice in groins and axillae.

  Cold, wet sheets or wet sponging (use wetting agent, e.g. cetrimide and fan).

  Surface cooling may be ineffective due to peripheral vasoconstriction. Therefore droperidol 5 mg IV used to produce vasodilatation.

  Consider cooling by gastric lavage or peritoneal dialysis with iced saline.

- Correct metabolic acidosis with at least 100 mmol $NaHCO_3$. Repeat as necessary.

  Correct raised K^+ with 50 ml of 50% dextrose +10 units soluble insulin.

If arrhythmias severe then see arrhythmia protocol.

An inotrope may be required to maintain cardiac output.

- When adequately rehydrated (as assessed by CVP and haematocrit) maintain adequate urinary output (with diuretic, if necessary). Each vial of dantrolene contains 3 g mannitol.

- Body temperature may be unstable for 24–48 h.

- After acute episode hypokalaemia, myoglobinuria.

- DIC may require treatment, assess clotting screen.

- Admit to ICU.

Later

- Repeat creatinine kinase after 24 h.

- Consider other diagnoses: thyroid crisis, salicylate toxicity, myopathy and recreational drugs – ecstasy, neuroleptic malignant syndrome.

- Refer patient and family for counselling about the implications of MH and to carry an alert card.

Note

- Vials of dantrolene contain 20 mg dantrolene sodium and 3 g mannitol, which require 60 ml of water to reconstitute (pH 9.5 ml). An average adult will initially require 200–250 ml.

If the episode has been controlled and surgery is essential, use a safe technique: regional block with plain bupivacaine or thiopentone, pancuronium and fentanyl, avoid suxamethonium and all volatile agents.

Malignant Hyperpyrexia

- Follow up patient and family.

Help line: St James's University Hospital trust (0113 206 5274, fax: 0113 206 4140).

Hot line bleep or 0525 420; out of office hours: 0345 333111.

Management of a patient known to be susceptible to MH

- Offer LA technique if possible.

- Discuss with regional centre results of muscle test and possible triggers.

- Clear theatre and all possible anaesthetic and resuscitation apparatus of all volatile agents.

- The likely triggers to avoid are suxamethonium and volatile anaesthetic agents but many other drugs and stress have been implicated as a cause.

- A safe technique could be a LA, ester or amide, with thiopentone, propofol, ketamine, nitrous oxide, midazolam, phenothiazines, opioids, non-depolarising muscle relaxants except tubocurare and reversal agents.

- Consider giving dantrolene 4 mg/kg for 24 h preoperatively, in 3 or 4 doses.

- Monitor all vital signs especially temperature, inspired and expired oxygen and carbon dioxide, ECG and oxygen saturation.

- Have available a surface cooling technique.

- Dantolene available.

Notes

- An early sign of hyperpyrexia is a low oxygen saturation on the pulse oximeter and a low oxygen concentration in the inspiratory limb of a circle absorber circuit due to a high oxygen consumption.

- Oxygen consumption can be calculated, in a steady state, from $X = F_o - C(V - F)/10VF$, where X = inspiratory oxygen concentration, F_o = fresh gas oxygen concentration, C = oxygen consumption in ml/min, V = ventilation l/min, F = fresh gas flow in l/min. Inspired oxygen concentration is obtained from the oxygen analysed in the inspiratory limb. The amount that this differs from the fresh gas oxygen concentration gives a measure of oxygen consumption.[2]

- A 17-year-old, 60 kg patient required 6 mg/kg of dantrolene. A dose of 2–3 mg/kg will usually be sufficient although 10 mg/kg has been used and repeated.[3] Some would routinely give an initial dose of 10 mg/kg.

- A circle breathing circuit with carbon dioxide absorption is usually recommended in MH. Most anaesthetic ventilators and circuits will not deliver a minute volume over 30 l/min. A higher minute volume will be obtained by letting the patient breath spontaneously using a non-rebreathing circuit and 100% oxygen if they are not paralysed. If carbon dioxide is not being eliminated it may be advisable to allow the patient to breath spontaneously.

References

1. Hopkins PM. Malignant hyperpyrexia: advances in clinical management and diagnosis. *British Journal of Anaesthesia* 2000; **85:** 118–28.
2. Philpott I. Malignant hyperpyrexia and oxygen consumption. *Anaesthesia and Intensive Care* 1990; **18:** 422–3.
3. Cain AG, Bell AD. How much dantrolene? A case of fulminating malignant hyperthermia. *Anaesthesia and Intensive Care* 1989; **17:** 500–9.

M

Nasoduodenal Tube

- A fine bore tube can be given rigidity by placing it in a freezer.

- It is easier to pass an oesophageal tube if the patient is given water to swallow at the same time as the tube is pushed forward. The water can be aspirated once the tube is in place.

- The correct placement of a nasogastric tube or fine bore feeding tube can be confirmed by (a) listening with a stethoscope over the stomach while insufflating with air; (b) aspiration of bile stained fluid; (c) radiography; (d) capnograph to exclude a tube in the airways.

- Erythromycin is a motilin agonist and gastrointestinal prokinetic agent; 200 mg IV causes antral contraction which facilitates the introduction of a fine bore feeding tube into the duodenum and beyond. ECG monitoring is advisable as IV erythromycin can produce serious cardiac arrhythmias.[1]

Nausea and Vomiting

> Reduce PONV.
>
> Choose a regional technique.
>
> Avoid fasting, hypotension and much movement.
>
> Consider IV fluids, nasogastric tube, propofol, oxygen.

Postoperative nausea and vomiting (PONV) is common but rarely life threatening. It frequently affects children and women, and patients having surgery on the middle ear and gynaecological procedures. The problem has importance because it is unpleasant and prevents day patients going home.

Causes

- *Predisposition.* Previous PONV, travel sickness, migraine.[2,3]

- *CNS.* Hypoxia, hypotension, middle and inner ear stimulation, raised intracranial pressure.

- *Drugs.* Antibiotics, ergometrine, opioids, nitrous oxide.

- *Altered GI function.* Ileus due to infection, handling of the bowel, fear, pain.

- Swallowed air and blood.

- *Metabolic.* Uraemia, liver failure, hypercalcaemia (osteolytic tumours), hypoglycaemia.

- *Starvation.* Increased volume and acidity of stomach secretions, hypoglycaemia.

- Bowel obstruction.

Avoidance

- Use a local anaesthetic technique.

- If GA consider IV infusion of crystalloid, propofol infusion, avoid nitrous oxide which will distend the bowel, avoid blowing gas into the stomach, nasogastric tube for several hours postoperatively.

Treatment[4]

- Reassure patient that nausea is not inevitable.

- Anxiolytic with amnesic premedication.

- Prokinetic drug preoperatively; metoclopramide 10 mg effective for some, domperidone 10 mg tablets.

- Postoperatively remain still and flat.

- IV fluids for hydration and mild hyperglycaemia.

- Nasogastric tube 10–12 Fg until no vomiting.

- Oxygen 2–3 l/min.

- Postoperative pain relief with local anaesthetic. If using a PCA, give antiemetic regularly.

Specific treatments

- Propofol for induction or total intravenous anaesthesia.

- Cholinergic antagonist for opioids. Atropine 600 μg, hyoscine 400 μg, cyclizine 50 mg.

- Serotonin antagonist: if excessive serotonin release in GI tract e.g. chemotherapy, ischaemia, infection.

- Phenothiazines: beware excess sedation, dysphoria, extrapyramidal movements, and particularly dystonia in children. Prochlorperazine is available as buccal tablets.

- Dexamethasone high dose 8 mg.

- Acupuncture at P6 point at wrist.

- Various herbal remedies, ginger.

- No one treatment has proven to be superior to any other.

Nerve Stimulators

A nerve stimulator for monitoring neuromuscular blockade transcutaneously produces 10–150 mA.

A stimulator to locate a nerve should give a current of 0.25–0.5 mA. A current over 1 mA applied to a nerve is painful. Nerve stimulators with no output control are not suitable for detecting nerves.

Polarity of electrodes

- The negative (cathode) terminal is used for nerve stimulation and localisation.[5]

- The cathode generates a depolarising current that excites the nerve fibre, whereas an anodal current makes the nerve fibre more resistant to excitation than normal. At the wrist the active negative electrode should be placed over the ulnar nerve for maximal twitch.[6]

- When locating a nerve through the skin the voltage in front of the tip of an uninsulated needle is greater than in an insulated needle. A nerve is most likely to be stimulated when it lies within a steep voltage gradient. This means that a nerve is most likely to be stimulated by an uninsulated needle when in front of the needle tip. With the insulated needle the nerve is likely to be stimulated when it is adjacent to the needle tip. So an uninsulated needle is safer for performing blocks as it is less likely to damage the nerve. The nerve will be stimulated before it is reached by the needle tip.[7]

- An inadequate stimulation current may lead to an overestimation of the degree of neuromuscular blockade. The minimum stimulus for the ulnar nerve at the wrist is at least 20 mA or 2.75 times the current needed to elicit the first detectable twitch.[8,9]

Assessing neuromuscular function after operation

- The head lift test is popular but does not correlate well with the response to the train of four (TOF) stimulus.[10] An arm lift for over 45, or better 60 s, correlates well with inspiratory force[11] and is better than testing head lift.

- TOF, four pulses at 2 Hz, are usually applied to the ulnar nerve at the wrist, to produce contraction of the hypothenar muscles, two lumbricals on the ulnar side, the interossei muscles and the adductor of the thumb. A non–depolarising block reduces the number of contractions: four twitches indicates complete recovery; three twitches 25% recovery and reversal can be given; two twitches indicates 20% recovery and one twitch 10% recovery and reversal should not be attempted. The TOF ratio is the force of the fourth twitch divided by the first twitch. The ratio can be difficult to judge so a double burst stimulus was introduced. This is one burst of three stimuli at 50 Hz followed after 0.75 s by two or three stimuli at 50 Hz. The second response should be at least 70% of the first before reversing the block.

- The force of contraction of adductor pollucis muscle can be monitored by attaching the tip of the thumb to a small syringe filled with 3 ml saline connected to a standard transducer system. The contraction is displayed on screen. If multiple readings are made the trace may not return to baseline and the system requires re-zeroing.[12]

- A pressure detector can be made by removing the air from a 250 ml IV fluid bag which is connected through IV tubing to a pressure transducer. The bag is placed in the palm of the closed hand. The hand and bag are wrapped securely with roll gauze. Nerve stimulator electrodes are placed on the ulnar nerve at the elbow. The motor response to ulnar nerve stimulation is seen as a pressure change recorded by the transducer.[13]

- When limb access is limited the temporal branch of the facial nerve can be stimulated. Or the accessory nerve can be stimulated by placing electrodes over the depression between the ramus of the mandible and the mastoid process or sternomastoid muscle. The nerve is stimulated as it passes deep to the styloid process and digastric.[14]

- Electrodes placed inferior and posterior to the medial malleolus of the tibia or below the sustentaculum tali will stimulate the posterior tibial nerve to give plantar flexion of the toes.[15]

- Recovery can be hastened by fluid loading to increase the volume for distribution and fluid flux at the neuromuscular junction.

Recovery

An anaesthetist volunteered to be partially paralysed, with a T_1–T_4 ratio of $1:0.2 = 0.2$. While supine the limbs could not be lifted, the tongue lay limp in the throat but without choking. The eyes would not focus and an inability to speak was due to not being able to lift the lips off the teeth. Once turned onto the side the arms could be moved easily in the plane of the bed. The lips moved to speak and the eyes focused. It is suggested that lying supine the muscles had to move against gravity, whereas on the side gravity was removed and function improved.[16]

Reflexes

- Patients are often hyo-reflexic immediately after anaesthesia.

- Diplopia and squint may be due to a sixth nerve weakness which occurs after anaesthesia and illness.

- Apnoea and vagal effects are produced by a variety of stimuli.

- Nasal irritation may cause apnoea, laryngeal closure bradycardia and vasovagal symptoms.[17] Parasympathetic innervation of the nose is not vagal but a derivative of the facial nerve travelling from the pons to the sphenopalatine ganglion through the facial nerve and then the greater superficial petrosal nerve and vidian nerve.[18]

- Vomiting and pain from pinnaplasty are reduced by blocking the auricula-temporal nerve supply to the ear by infiltrating local anaesthetic over the posterior aspect of the zygoma, anterior to the external auditory meatus. Then blocking the greater auricular nerve by infiltration of the cervical plexus at the mid-point of the posterior border of the sternomastoid.

- Both the muscles of the eye and the muscles of the ear seem to be part of an emetic reflex.[19]

Nerve Damage during Surgery

- The facial nerve and terminal branches of the trigeminal nerve are damaged by pressure to the face and around the eyes.

- The brachial plexus can be damaged by traction whenever the arm is abducted, or the head pulled laterally.

- The radial nerve is at risk from compression as it curves around the humerus.

- The ulnar nerve is exposed in the ulnar grove of the humerus. The ulnar nerve may be damaged by compression in the cubital tunnel as it passes from the arm to forearm. When the forearm is pronated the cubital tunnel is in contact with any flat surface and can be at risk from compression. Supination of the forearm rotates the elbow such that the cubital tunnel is no longer in contact with any flat surface and is a safer position to fix the forearm in, when attaching it to a supporting board.[20]

- Lithotomy may damage the sciatic or femoral nerves.

- The lateral popliteal nerve is exposed to pressure as it curves around the head of the fibula.

- The ligaments, muscles and discs of the spine can be stretched in lithotomy.

References

1. Weekes JWN. Erythromycin to facilitate placement of naso-duodenal feeding tubes. *Anaesthesia and Intensive Care* 1994; **22:** 318.

2. Toner CC et al. Prediction of postoperative nausea and vomiting using a logistic regression model. *British Journal of Anaesthesia* 1996; **76:** 347–51.

3. Palazzo M, Evans R. Logistic regression analysis of fixed patient factors for postoperative sickness: a model for risk assessment. *British Journal of Anaesthesia* 1993; **70:** 135–40.

4. Palazzo MG, Strunin L. Anaesthesia and emesis. *Canadian Anaesthetists Society Journal* 1984; **31:** 407–15.

5. Tulchinsky A, Weller RS, Rosenblum M. Nerve stimulator polarity and brachial plexus block. *Anesthesia and Analgesia* 1993; **77:** 100–3.

6. Berger JJ, Gravenstein JS, Munson ES. Electrode polarity and peripheral nerve stimulation. *Anesthesiology* 1982; **56:** 402–4.

7. Jones RP, De Jonge M, Smith BE. Voltage fields surrounding needles used in regional anaesthesia. *British Journal of Anaesthesia* 1992; **68:** 515–18.

8. Sois MB. Train-of-four ratio is not always independent of stimulating current. *Anesthesiolgy* 1990; **73:** 573–5.

9. Lawson D. Doctor are you sure the patient is paralysed? *Anesthesiolgy* 1990; **73:** 574.

10. Bar ZG. The arm lift test. *Anaesthesia* 1985; **40:** 630–3

11. Viby-Mogensen J, Jorgensen BC, Ording H. Residual curarisation in the recovery room. *Anesthesiology* 1979; **50:** 539–41.

12. Moretti EA, Cardoso R, Rafizadeh M. A simple device to monitor neuromuscular blockade. *Anesthesia and Analgesia* 1991; **72:** 563–4.

13. Smith SB, Grenawalt JW. A simple technique for remote monitoring of neuromuscular blockade. *Anesthesiology* 1986; **65:** 562.

14. Meakin G. Stimulation of the spinal accessory nerve as a method of monitoring neuromuscular transmission. *Anaesthesia* 1993; **48:** 85.

15. Frank LP. But where will I put my twitch monitor? *Anesthesia and Analgesia* 1986; **65:** 425.

16. Hans P et al. Reversal of neurological deficit with naloxone: an additional report. *Intensive Care Medicine* 1992; **18:** 362–3.

17. Rice ASC. Peripheral nerve damage and regional anaesthesia. *British Journal of Anaesthesia* 1995; **75:** 116.

18. Prosser DP. Adaptation of an intravenous cannula for paediatric regional anaesthesia. *Anaesthesia* 1996; **51:** 510.

19. Sarnat AJ. A simple device for testing peripheral nerve stimulators. *Anesthesiology* 1984; **61:** 624–5.

20. Stoelting RK. Postoperative ulnar nerve palsy – is it a preventable complication? *Anesthesia and Analgesia* 1993; **76:** 7–9.

Obstetrics

Labour is established when contractions are regular and painful with

- either membranes ruptured spontaneously or a show;
- cervix effaced.

Management of normal labour[1]

- Sips of water or ice.
- There is an ileus and no food should be taken.
- Dehydration give IV fluids. The normal serum sodium is low in pregnancy so care is required not to dilute the plasma sodium further with dextrose solutions.
- Entonox for pain on admission, during examinations and in the second stage. Start self-administered Entonox before a series of contractions.

Ante-acid therapy

- Ranitidine 150 mg orally every 6 h
- Elective caesarean section 150 mg oral ranitidine 3 h preoperatively and 0.3 M sodium citrate 30 ml before theatre.
- Emergency section 50 mg IV ranitidine and 0.3 M sodium citrate 30 ml before theatre.

Oxytocics: 1 ml syntometrine = ergometrine 0.5 mg with oxytocin 5 units IM.

A Partogram or record of labour should include

a) *Foetal condition.* Foetal heart rate (FHR) and pattern, colour of amniotic fluid – clear or meconium staining.

b) *Progress of labour.* Cervical dilatation. Spontaneous labour primigravida 1.9 ± 1.2 cm/h; multigravida 3.5 ± 2.7 cm/h.

Descent of foetal head. 5/5 above brim, 4/5 entering brim, 3/5 above brim, 2/5 head engaged, 1/5 sinciput tipped abdominally, 0/5 engaged.[2]

c) *Maternal condition.* BP, HR, temperature, urine output.

Foetal heart rate patterns

Normal

1. Rate 120–160 beats/min, no change with contractions, baseline variation <5 beats/min.

2. Bradycardia: 100–120 beats/min, no change with contractions, baseline variation 5 beats/min or more – *a foetus with a good vagal tone.*

3. Acceleration of FHR at start of contraction and return to baseline before or just after contraction – *good reflex reactivity of foetus circulation.*

4. Early deceleration of FHR starts with onset of contraction, rate returns to baseline by end of contraction, deceleration does not exceed 40 beats/min – *good progress.*

Suspicious patterns

1. Variable decelerations show decrease FHR at onset or early in contraction, deceleration has irregular shape, variability usually >50 beats/min.

2. Baseline 120–160 beats/min, baseline variability 5 beats or more per minute, it may precede more abnormal patterns.

3. Baseline tachycardia 160–180 beats/min, baseline variability 5 beats/min or more, no change with contraction, patterns may be secondary to maternal pyrexia or ketosis.

4. Loss of baseline variability. Baseline FHR variability of 5 beats/min or less. The less

Obstetrics

the baseline variability the greater the possibility of foetal asphyxia. Loss of baseline variability may be secondary to maternal drugs – sedatives and analgesics.

Abnormal patterns

1. Late decelerations. Any deceleration with the lowest point past the peak of contraction. Usually – hypoxia. Greater the lag time the more serious the hypoxia.

2. Complicated loss of baseline variability. Baseline variability of less than 5 beats/min with abnormal baseline and/or accelerations.

3. Complicated tachycardia >160 beats/min plus deceleration with loss of baseline variability. Measure foetal pH – under 7.25 is abnormal.

Maternal causes: supine hypotension, ketosis, uterine hyperactivity.

Epidural in labour

Indications

- Request by mother for pain relief and consent.

- To reduce the maternal work of labour in diabetes, hypertension and pre-eclampsia, cardiac, respiratory and other diseases.

- To protect the foetus: prematurity, breech and multiple pregnancies. Any foetus at risk from hypoxia or sedative drugs.

- Operative procedures, intrauterine death.

- Uterine scar: allows assessment of the progress of the labour and scar.

Absolute and relative contraindications

- Maternal refusal, difficult anatomy, clotting deficiency, neurological disease, potential or actual massive loss of blood, e.g. placenta praevia or abruption, sepsis.

Preparation

Tilt to prevent aorto-caval compression, IV fluids and vasoconstrictors to prevent hypotension.

After each dose monitor maternal BP and pulse with FHR every 5 min for 30 min, then for every 30 min.

For inadequate block

- avoid injecting air or saline into epidural space, which can pocket around a nerve root, when testing for loss of resistance. Second dose will get rid of this pain.

- add local anaesthetic volume; groin pain may indicate ovarian pain from renal axis referred to groin.

- consider second catheter if first fails or partially works.

Shivering due to vasodilatation and central cooling or local anaesthetic toxicity.

Ambulatory epidural

A combination of low concentration local anaesthetic and a lipid soluble opioid can give pain relief without a dense motor block.

A regime of an initial epidural dose of 15 ml 0.1% bupivacaine (or ropivacaine 1%) with fentanyl 2 μg/ml, with topup of 10 ml by doctor or PCA (lockout 30 min) administration has been used.[3] There is no benefit in giving additional drugs into the CSF but they may cause meningism.[4]

Massive haemorrhage – see blood transfusion

- Monitor BP, HR, CVP (if time permits), urine output.

- Fibrinogen <1 g/l and bleeding give cryoprecipitate 10 bags = 2 g fibrinogen. Platelets $<50 \times 10^9$/l give platelets.

- APH live baby LSCS. Dead baby rupture membranes, stimulate labour, pain relief, check clotting.

- PPH ergometrine 0.5 mg, biamanual compression of uterus. Carboprost IV 250 µg to 1 mg effective in 3 min.

Pre-eclamptic toxaemia

- Proteinuria >500 mg urinary protein in 24 h, BP 150/100 or over.

- Imminent eclampsia if persistent headache, nausea and vomiting, epigastric pain, visual disturbance, oliguria, restlessness, muscle twitching, hyper-reflexia.

- Treatment: aim for BP 140/90 or less, prevent convulsions, exclude coagulation defect, optimal analgesia, expedite delivery.

Hypertension treatment

- Hydralazine 50 mg in 50 ml 0.9% saline. Infuse 15 ml in first hour and then reduce by 5 ml/h. Caution large fall in BP and rise in HR.

- Diazemules 5–10 mg IV slowly and then infusion.

- Urine output frusemide 10–20 mg and repeat.

- Consider an epidural after test of coagulation normal.

Eclampsia

- Airway, breathing, oxygen, diazemules at least 10 mg, pethidine or epidural if coagulation normal.

- Magnesium sulphate. Loading dose 4 g IV over 15 min as 8 ml 50% solution in 50 ml 0.9% saline. Then 1–2 g/h, as 5 g in 50 ml 0.9% saline. Continue for 24 h after the last fit with a reducing dose. Or give a single dose of 4 g IV and 3 g IM to each buttock.

- Monitor: ECG, pulse oximeter, FHR, patellar reflexes, respiratory rate and urine output >25 ml/h.

- Magnesium serum levels: normal 0.7–1.0 mmol/l, 2–4 mmol/l therapeutic, 5 mmol/l patellar reflexes go, 6 mmol/l striated muscle relaxed and respiratory depression with respiratory arrest at 7.5 mmol/l. Cardiac arrest at 12 mmol/l.

- Relative contraindication for magnesium: heart block, myasthenia gravis.

HELLP syndrome

Haemolysis, elevated liver enzymes and low platelets, high risk of morbidity. Often a complication of pre-eclampsia, but some mothers have only mild hypertension or no significant proteinuria.

At risk from intravascular coagulation, thromboembolism, abruptio placenta, renal failure, pulmonary oedema and ruptured liver haematoma.

Outcome is influenced by the severity of the hypertension and the gestational age.[5,6]

Diabetic mother

- Diabetic regime of IV dextrose, potassium and insulin with epidural analgesia to reduce the work of labour and to aid the delivery of a large dysmature baby. Monitor glucose in mother at least every 3 h during labour; mother and baby at least every 3 h post delivery.

- Examine baby for congenital abnormalities, hypoglycaemia, RDS.

DVT prophylaxis enoxaparin 20 mg SC.

- Heparin does not cross the placenta barrier and does not affect the foetus but it should be discontinued during labour.

Amniotic fluid embolism (high mortality)

Consider if unexplained cyanosis and hypoxia or hypotension.

117

Obstetrics

O

Maintain oxygenation: if in doubt intubate and ventilate as RDS and DIC may develop.

CVS function: support with inotropes.

Renal function: measure urine output, treat renal failure.

One-Lung Anaesthesia

Double lumen tubes

- The whole of the right lung is better ventilated from a left bronchial tube which does not obstruct the right upper lobe bronchus wherever it arises.

- Pass the tube with the concave distal section anteriorly, once this is in the trachea, rotate the tube 90° so that the concavity is towards the bronchus to be intubated.

- The fibre-optic scope is recommended as an introducer and to verify the position of the tube in relation to the carina and to each bronchus.

- Once in place the tracheal cuff is inflated and leaks are detected by noise at the mouth and a difference between inspired and expired gas volumes.

- Inflation of each bronchial cuff is tested by clamping the gas flow from the breathing circuit to one side of the double lumen tube and opening the suction port on that side. If the bronchial cuff is inflated no ventilation should occur in the clamped side and no tidal volume should be lost. The compliance will decrease while one lung is ventilated and the ventilator pressure may need to be adjusted to maintain the minute volume.

- A urinary catheter inserted down one lumen of the double lumen tube can enable one-lung anaesthesia to continue when the double lumen tube has failed

to separate the two lungs. Passing the catheter down the side on which the lung should be deflated and distending the balloon will collapse that lung. Passing a catheter down the side to be inflated and connecting to a ventilator can be useful if the cuff on the bronchial tube fails.[7]

- In small adults and children endobronchial blockade can be performed using a tracheal tube, a fibre-optic bronchoscope adapter and a 6 Fr Fogerty catheter. It is difficult to provide an airtight seal when the Fogerty catheter is introduced and manipulated. BD syringes are supplied with a rubber cap which fits the orifice of the bronchocath adapter. A hole is made in it with a large needle and the catheter will pass through making an airtight seal.[8]

Continuous positive airway pressure (CPAP)

- Reduces the shunt through the non-ventilated lung.

- CPAP to the non-ventilated lung during one-lung anaesthesia can be provided by using a 1 l reservoir bag connected to a Portex Y-shaped connector 100/277/000 to which oxygen is connected. This is then connected to a second Portex Y connector 100/276/000 which fits to lumen to the non-ventilated lung. This side tube is fitted with a length of tubing, which causes resistance and creates the positive pressure. The airway pressure depends on the fresh gas flow and the resistance of the tubing. A manometer is added to measure the pressure.[9]

- An Ayre's T piece can be connected to the non-ventilated lung with a fresh gas flow of oxygen. The distal end is connected to an exhaust valve, reservoir bag and a pressure gauge. The valve is adjusted to give the appropriate pressure.[10]

- The fresh gas inlet of the Bain circuit is connected to any oxygen source with a flowmeter and oxygen flow at 1–2 l/min. The circuit is connected to the non-ventilated lumen of the double lumen tube. The expiratory valve is set to give the desired CPAP which is read from a manometer[11] (Figure 39).

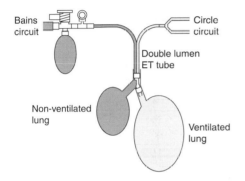

Figure 39 – Bains circuit to give CPAP to non-ventilated lung.

One-lung lavage

- Lavage is used in asthmatics to remove secretions, casts and toxic material from massive inhalation. The lavage fluid must be of sufficient volume to spread into the bronchioli but not toxic to the lung. A danger is the rapid absorption of solution affecting cardiac function. One solution is isotonic saline with serum concentrations of potassium and 10 mg/l hydrocortisone to reduce inflammation.

- Tubing containing this isotonic saline, heated to 37°C by passing through a Fenwal blood warmer, is placed in series with a water manometer which is then attached to the bronchial tube. The manometer pressure reading is kept at +30 cmH₂O by adjusting the height of the fluid bag[12,13] (Figure 40).

119

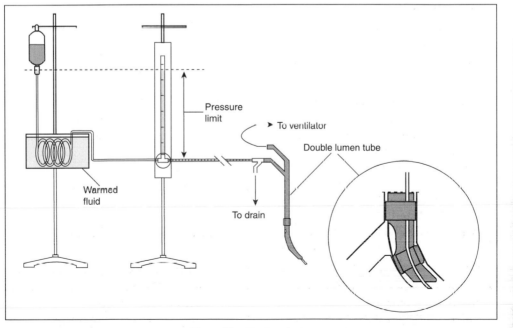

Figure 40 – One-lung lavage.

One-Lung Anaesthesia

Preoxygenation

- The value of preoxygenation is to prevent the normal adult P_aO_2 12.7 kPa on room air falling to 7.1 kPa after 2 min of apnoea.[14] Four vital capacity breaths of 100% oxygen are almost as effective as 3 min breathing from a Magill system. Maximum exhalation before breathing the oxygen improves oxygenation when four vital capacity breaths are taken. In order to deliver four vital capacity breaths a 4 l or two 2 l bags are needed in series.

- If four vital capacity breaths are used there must be a breathing circuit with a non-rebreathing valve, an adequate fresh gas reservoir using the oxygen flush if the bags collapse during inspiration, and a perfect seal.[15]

- Arterial oxygen tensions were measured in ten patients after 100% oxygen for four deep breaths and 100% oxygen with quiet breathing for 5 min. Only three out of the ten patients achieved a higher P_aO_2 after 5 min of 100% oxygen. In an emergency, four deep breaths of oxygen appreciably increases arterial oxygen tension.[16]

- If the patient has been preoxygenated with 100% oxygen and the oesophagus is then mistakenly intubated it may be 5–6 min before cyanosis occurs. Because of the lapse in time the anaesthetist may not link an oesophageal intubation with the cyanosis and look for other causes.[17]

- An alternative to the mask is a mouthpiece. This can be obtained from Ohmeda or improvised from the elbow connection of a breathing circuit placed between the lips.[18]

References

1. Steer P, Flint C. ABC of labour care. *British Medical Journal* 1999; **318**: 793–6.

2. Crichton D. A reliable method of establishing the level of fetal head in obstetrics. *South African Medical Journal* 1974; **48**: 784–7.

3. Murphy JD, Hendeson K, Bowden MI, Lewis M, Cooper GM. Bupivacaine versus bupivacaine plus fentanyl for epidural analgesia: effect on maternal satisfaction. *British Medical Journal* 1991; **302**: 564–7.

4. Price C, Lafreniere L, Brosnan C, Findley I. Regional analgesia in early active labour: combined spinal epidural vs epidural. *Anaesthesia* 1998; **53**: 951–5.

5. van Pampus MG et al. Maternal and perinatal outcome after expectant management of the HELLP syndrome compared with pre-eclampsia without HELLP syndrome. *European Journal of Obstertics and Gynaecology* 1998; **76**: 31–6.

6. Poole JH. Aggresive management of HELLP syndrome and eclampsia. *AACN Clinical Issues* 1997; **4**: 524–38.

7. Conacher ID. The urinary catheter as a bronchial blocker. *Anaesthesia* 1983; **38**: 475–7.

8. Ransom ES, Norfleet EA. Syringe cap prevents leaks during one-lung ventilation. *Anesthesia and Analgesia* 1995; **82**: 1538.

9. Galloway DW, Bowler GMR. A simple CPAP system during one-lung anaesthesia. *Anaesthesia* 1988; **43**: 708–9.

10. Thiagarajah S. A device for applying CPAP to the non-ventilated upper lung during one-lung ventilation. *Anesthesiology* 1984; **60**: 253–4.

11. Scheler MS, Varvel JR. CPAP oxygenation during one-lung ventilation using a Bain circuit. *Anesthesiology* 1987; **66**: 708.

12. Spalitta JT, Marino RJ. More on one-lung lavage. *Anesthesiology* 1983; **59**: 166.

13. Spragg RG, Benumof JF, Alfrey DD. New methods for performance of unilateral lung lavage. *Anesthesiology* 1982; **57**: 535–9.

14. Lawes EG. The need for oxygenation prior to tracheal intubation. *Anaesthesia* 1985; **40**: 588–9.

15. McCrory JW, Matthews JNS. Comparison of four methods of preoxygenation. *British Journal of Anaesthesia* 1990; **64**: 571–6.

16. Sellers WFS, Rhodin A. Pre-oxygenation. *British Journal of Anaesthesia* 1985; **57**: 1268–9.

17. Howells TH. A hazard of pre-oxygenation. *Anaesthesia* 1985; **40**: 86.

18. Keifer RB, Strit JA. Preoxygenation. *Anesthesiology* 1995; **83**: 429.

Pacemakers

Check preoperatively

- Reason for use: heart block with ischaemia or infarction, syncope attacks.

- Types of pacemaker. NBG Code: 1: chamber paced (A atrium, V ventricle, D dual); 2: chamber sensed AVD; 3: response to sensing ('T triggered, I inhibited, D dual, R reverse); 4: programmability and 5: functions available in tachycardia. Date: it was fitted and last checked. If over 1 year since last check consider recheck. Lithium batteries last 5–10 years.

- Evidence of malfunction: syncope, dizziness, palpitations, chest pain, dyspnoea, orthopnoea, oedema, abnormal ECG.

- Check ECG, urea and electrolytes.

Diathermy

- Bipolar is preferred as the current is limited to the space between the tips of the forceps.

- Unipolar diathermy plate and probe should be 15 cm away from the pacemaker and its wires. The current field should not cross the pacemaker and its wires.

Check

- Isoprenaline and transcutaneous pacemaker available, programme pacer to VOO (asynchronous mode).

- Monitor ECG, pulse oximeter, avoid hypoxia and hypotension (give a fluid preload especially if dehydrated).

- Remember patient has a limited/fixed cardiac output and may not compensate for blood loss or vasodilation.

Pain

Pain can be classified as acute and chronic; nociceptive, neurogenic, sympathetic and emotional.

- *Nociceptive pain* is associated with tissue damage. It is well localised, aggravated by movement, relieved by rest.

Treatment of nociceptive pain

- NSAIDs and opioids.

- *Neurogenic pain* is associated with nerve damage e.g. phantom pain, post-herpetic neuralgia, trigeminal neuralgia, pressure on a nerve and peripheral neuropathy. Features include: allodynia – a non-painful stimulus is felt as pain; hyperaesthesia – a little pain is felt as extreme pain; dysaesthesia – abnormal sensation. The damage may be peripheral, in the spinal cord or in the central nervous system as in a CVA.

Treatment of neurogenic pain

- Amitriptyline, and some other tricyclic antidepressant, are effective in sub-anti-depressant doses e.g. amitriptyline 10 mg. Various anticonvulsants: carbamazepine for trigeminal neuralgia, sodium valproate, gabapentin >1.8 g daily.

- *Sympathetic pain* is deep in the tissues and poorly localised. There may be signs of a disturbance of the sympathetic nervous system, ischaemia, coldness, oedema, abnormal sweating. The term complex regional pain syndrome (CRPS) is sub divided into type 1 with trauma and type 2 with obvious peripheral nerve damage.

Treatment of sympathetic pain

- Sometimes, but not always, a sympathetic block will relieve the pain. Causalgia (CRPS type 2) due to a gunshot wound is a pain syndrome often relieved by sympathetic blockade.

121

- *Emotional pain* is a symptom of depression, grief, anxiety, inability to cope and fear. Consider the meaning of words such as heartache and a pain in the neck. If pain is present in normal tissue consider either referred or emotional pain.

Treatment of emotional pain

- Do not give drugs of dependency for emotional pain.

- Analgesics that give pain relief for short periods of 30–60 min are likely to lead to dependency.

- Counselling, pain management program.

Strategy for pain relief (Table 5)

- Non-drug: explanation and relief of anxiety, relaxation and suggestion, acupuncture, stimulation to produce an inhibitory descending spinal stimulus by transcutaneous stimulation, heat, cold, spinal cord stimulation.

- Drugs: NSAIDs, opioids, amitriptyline, carbamazepine, sodium valproate, gabapentine and sodium channel membrane stabilisers. Muscle relaxants clonazepam, diazepam, baclofen,

dantrolene, botulinum toxin. Others: steroids, mood enhancing drugs. Nerve blocks with local anaesthetic, heat lesions, cryotherapy, alcohol, phenol and surgery.

Acute postoperative pain relief

Treatment: Balanced pain relief: NSAIDs, opioids and local anaesthetic in appropriate doses reduce the side effects of any one drug given alone.

NSAIDs inhibit cyclo-oxygenase and so prevent the conversion of arachadonic acid to prostaglandin.

NSAIDs[1]

- not sufficient alone for major surgery,

- decrease opioid requirements and side effects,

- enhance opioid analgesia,

- increase bleeding time and may increase blood loss,

- recommended for day cases.

NSAIDs considerations

- Many drug interactions to be aware of.

Table 5 – Strategy for pain relief

Non-drug	Drugs	Nerve blocks
Explanation	NSAIDs	Local or regional anaesthesia
Relief of fear/anxiety	Weak opioid	Radiofrequency lesions
Distraction	Strong opioids	Cryotherapy
Relaxation	Neurogenic pain: amitriptyline,	Glycerol
Suggestion/hypnosis	carbamazepine, sodium valproate,	Alcohol
Acupuncture 3–10 Hz	gabapentin and ketamine	Phenol
TENS 80–100 Hz	Muscle relaxants: Diazepam,	Surgery
"close gate" stimulation	Baclofen, Dantrolene, Botulinum	Dorsal root entry zone lesions
with heat, cold, rubbing	toxin	
Dorsal column stimulation	Membrane stabilizers	
	Sodium channel inhibition	
	Spinal clonidine	
	Steroids	
	Sympathetic block	
	Guanethidine, Debrisoquine	

- Not recommended if increased bleeding, pre-eclamptic toxaemia or uncontrolled hypertension, aspirin sensitive asthma particularly with nasal polyps in adults.

- Intramuscular diclofenac should be avoided due to muscle destruction and pain.

- Tell patients about rectal drugs before use.

- Use with care and monitor urine production in renal failure. Prostaglandins promote renal vasodilatation.

- Monitor renal function postoperatively.

- Use with care in elderly, diabetes, vascular disease, after cardiac, hepatobiliary and renal or vascular surgery.

- Do not give aspirin to children under 12 years (Reye's syndrome).

Opioids

- Morphine acts as a mu receptor agonist. Others act at sigma and kappa receptors.

Side effects often limit use:

- Nausea and vomiting. Give anticholinergic antiemetic.

- Constipation due to smooth muscle spasm. Give regular laxative after several days of use.

- Hallucinations delusions and dysphoria. Give diazepam in small doses (2–5 mg).

- Reduce respiratory centre's sensitivity to carbon dioxide so arterial P_aCO_2 higher than the normal 5.3 kPa. Reduce ability to respond to a carbon dioxide challenge. In excess respiratory failure. Give naloxone 400 µg or doxapram 20–100 mg IV.

- If morphine dose is increasing without pain relief consider (a) patient only getting a mood change, (b) patient producing an excess of M3G which is inhibiting the morphine effect. In both cases reduce the morphine dose.

Postoperative pain relief

- Assessment of pain is the key to good pain relief. If it is not measured and recorded it will not be treated.

- *Mild pain*. Oral NSAIDs and weak opioids such as codeine and dextropropoxyphene. Local anaesthetic block.

- *Strong pain*. Combination of NSAIDs, opioids and local anaesthetic blocks.

- Give analgesics regularly, not as needed.

- Opioid – morphine either 1–2 mg IV in patient controlled device, lockout 5–10 min, or offer 0.15 mg/kg every 1 h intramuscularly.

- Never give intramuscular analgesics if patient is vasoconstricted, hypovolaemia or in severe pain.

- Patients receiving high dose opioids such as slow release morphine for cancer or addiction and fentanyl patches should:

  - continue their regime or convert to systemic doses by halving the oral dose. Then add extra opioid for pain relief.

  - monitor respiration particularly after a LA block. Pain is a stimulus to respiration. LA block will remove pain and apnoea may follow. Fentanyl patches have an effect for 48 h and apnoea may occur long after the LA block is established or topped up.

PCA

- Check: dose, concentration, lockout period, dose limit in a set number of hours if used, one-way valve to stop IV. Line filling with drug if cannula blocked, antisyphon device.

- Safety: Prefilled syringe to avoid errors in preparation, label syringe, lock syringe in place, check programme, lock programme. Nurse should record vital signs, pain and sedation score and check the injection site. Additional prescriptions for antiemetic, naloxone and NSAID. All staff should have training in the use of the device.

- A continuous infusion becomes nurse controlled analgesia with additional training and responsibilities.

- A continuous infusion, in addition to a normal PCA dose, is appropriate for the patient already receiving opioids for cancer pain or drug addiction. The 24 h oral dose of morphine should be halved to convert to the 24 h IV or IM dose.

- It is not good practice to mix drugs in the same syringe, giving more of one increases the amount of the other. Take two syringes.

Pain in children

Children experience pain as much as adults. They should receive analgesics in appropriate doses by weight and need.

- Chart facial expression, body movement and abdominal respiration. Each scored 0 = no pain, 1 = mild pain, 2 = severe pain, will guide prescribing with a score of 2 indicating the need for analgesia. This score can be used in conjunction with a sedation score.[2]

- Scales to assess pain in children can be made in many ways. There are vertical scales as in ladder rungs, monkey on a pole, and horizontal scales such as happy to crying faces.

- Children 3–7 years find a horizontal abacus more interesting. Children 8–14 find the vertical monkey and pole more interesting but the horizontal scale better represents their understanding of the concept of increasing pain.[3]

- To assess the effectiveness of a local anaesthetic block, particularly in children, a 50 ml intravenous bag, filled with 30 ml air, is connected to an aneroid pressure

gauge. The bag is placed over the incision site and pressure is applied to the bag. The point of discomfort is recorded as a pressure, which is preferred to a pinprick, to assess the effectiveness of local anaesthesia.[4]

Alternative means of pain relief

- Inhaled analgesia. Self-administered Entonox for short procedures. The concept of inhalation analgesia dates back to 1866 in modern medicine and to the 12th century BC in antiquity.[5]

- Fentanyl is effective as an aerosol in doses of 100–300 μg but it is bitter as are most opioids.[6]

- Children with trauma pain respond well to 0.1 mg/kg diamorphine solution, given in not more than 0.1 ml to each nostril.

- A bolus of lidocaine 100 mg IV half an hour before skin incision, followed by an infusion of 2 mg/min for 24 h postoperatively acts as an analgesic.[7] The patients should be monitored for toxic effects of the local anaesthetic.

- Joint surgery; 1 mg of intra-articular morphine provides significant pain relief for 24 h but bupivacaine does not increase the benefit.[8]

- An alternative route for PCA or intermittent opiates is a subcutaneous or intramuscular indwelling catheter which reduces the pain of frequent injections. The cannula should be placed into the pectoral, deltoid, abdomen or thigh muscles. Diacetyl-morphine (heroine) is pain free to inject compared to morphine.[9]

- A bilateral infra-orbital nerve block using 1 ml of lidocaine 1% with epinephrine reduces the pain of cleft lip surgery.[10]

- Phantom limb pain can occur immediately following amputation but it can also re-appear and be precipitated by another event years later. A patient who previously experienced phantom limb pain, which had gone, had the same pain brought back by chemotherapy for another disease. The pain was controlled by a ketamine infusion starting with 10 mg/h.[11]

Painful stimuli to produce arousal

- Gentle pressure applied to the tragus, pushing it to cover the external meatus, will wake a sleeping patient without a startle. Squeezing the muscle belly of trapezius, at the base of the neck, between finger and thumb is painful and leaves no bruise.[12]

Pain in back due to surgery

- The incidence and severity of post-operative back pain can be reduced by placing a bag wedge to fill the lumbosacral curve and then inflating to 25 mmHg if the patient is supine and to 30 mmHg in the lithotomy position.[13]

Penile turgescence

- Penile turgescence can limit cystoscopy and other urological procedures. Various remedies have been suggested including: ketamine 0.5–2 mg/kg and/or physostigmine 1.5 mg, inhaled amylnitrate and topical nitroglycerin 2% paste.[14]

Poisoning

Management of poisoning

Assess: airway, breathing, circulation
If hypotensive give fluids and/or
 vasopressor at same time as intubation
 and ventilation
Protect airway from aspiration
Gastric washout if within 1 h of ingestion
Give activated charcoal: adult 50 g,
 child 25 g
Give antidote
IV fluid
BNF for toxicology telephone numbers

Protocol[15]

- Immediate management: assess airway, breathing, cardiac output. Intubation and IPPV may reduce the venous return and lead to a very low cardiac output. A vasoconstrictor, norepinephrine, and IV fluids should be in progress if hypotension exists before IPPV.

- Antidote where applicable.

- Activated charcoal, 50 g adult, 25 g child, should be instilled into the stomach up to 4–6 h after ingestion. Protect the airway first.

- Blood sample for toxicology, electrolytes and arterial blood gases.

- Twenty-four hour poison advice number in BNF.

- Gastric lavage is rarely indicated if more than 1 h has passed since ingestion.

Specific drugs and specific treatments

Ecstasy and other amphetamines[16]

- Effects: sympathetic overactivity, hyperpyrexia, rhabdomyolisis, muscle rigidity, reduced consciousness and fitting. Excessive drinking leads to water intoxication and hyponatraemia.

- Treatment: dantolene, cooling, control of acidosis, hypertonic saline, reduce cerebral oedema, maintain urine output, beta-blockade, sedation for fits.

Opiates[17]

- Effect: respiratory depression.

- Treatment: naloxone 1–10 mg bolus and then titrate dose by IV infusion.

Organophosphorus insecticides

- Effects: muscarinic effects of acetylcholine, paralysis, bradycardia, secretions, coma.

- Treatment: atropine 2 mg repeated, Pralidoxime mesylate within 24 h.

Paracetamol

- Effect: hepatocellular necrosis especially with alcohol.

- Treatment: acetylcysteine start 150 mg/kg in 200 ml glucose up to 24 h after ingestion and methionine start 2.5 g orally within 10 h of ingestion.

Tricyclic antidepressants[18]

- Effect: conduction delays in heart.

- Treatment: alkalinisation with sodium loading using hypertonic sodium bicarbonate and then isotonic saline. Do not give antiarrhythmics which further slow conduction. Refractory hypotension give norepinephrine.

Bowel irrigation

- Six children, aged 18 months to 5 years, who had ingested tricyclic antidepressants some hours before and where the drug was considered to be in the intestine were given polyethylene glycol sulphate via a nasogastric tube at 500 ml/h for 6 h or until the rectal effluent was clear. Plasma electrolytes were monitored throughout the treatment but did not change. A 67% reduction in drug absorption was found with whole bowel irrigation. This irrigation may be indicated when there is serious intoxication with potential loss of life providing that strict fluid balance is maintained and the airway is protected from aspiration.[19]

Porphyrias[20]

The Porphyrias are a group of diseases due to a congenital defect in haem synthesis.

Diagnosis: Identify susceptible individuals by family history and test blood and urine for products appropriate to the known possible variant. If there is no family history test for elevated activity of erythrocyte porphobilinogen (PBG), urine analysis for delta-aminolaevulinic acid (ALA) and PBG is less sensitive.

If the patient is having an acute attack test plasma, urine and stool for a porphyrin profile.

Administration of an anaesthetic

- Avoid starvation: Infuse saline–dextrose solutions with care to avoid hyponatraemia.

- Avoid barbiturates and etomidate: Propofol is probably safe or ketamine.

- Give phenothiazenes and with care diazepam or temazepam.

- LA blocks are safe but effect may be confused with concomitant neural effect of porphyria.

- Safe: Nitrous oxide, halothane, isoflurane, pancuronium and suxamethonium, opioids.

Full list in Ref. 20.

Pulse Oximeter

Probes

- The spring in the probe may become weak. To hold the probe the cut finger of a latex glove can be slipped over it once it is on the finger. The elasticity of the latex holds the probe in place.[21]

- A clip on probe can be positioned on the nasal septum, the lip or the tongue but may become contaminated. A 2–3 cm long piece of the finger of a vinyl glove fits over one arm of the probe. This finger stall acts to protect the probe and is disposed of after a single use.[22] The vinyl does not interfere with the pulse oximeter reading.[23]

- The pulse signal can be enhanced by inducing vasodilatation using: glyceryl trinitrate ointment to the finger; a disposable glove filled with warm water placed in the patient's hand for about 2 min.[24]

Signal

The pulse oximeter probe emits light of two wavelengths in the red and infra red range. The ratio of the amount of light absorbed at each wavelength is used to calculate the total haemoglobin and the reduced haemoglobin and hence the oxyhaemoglobin. Most of the light is absorbed by the tissues. To detect haemoglobin the device ignores all non-pulsed signals.

- Oximeters are designed to reject ambient light. When the ambient light intensity is high the photodetector may not be able to sense enough light transmitted through tissue to calculate a reliable oxygen saturation.[25]

- Two patients with a haemoglobin of less than 2.9 mmol/l (4.7 g/dl) had readings of SaO_2 99% and 97%. This suggests that the reading obtained even in severe anaemia gives a useful indicator of oxygen saturation.[26]

- The presence of methaemoglobin in blood will give a pulse oximeter reading towards 85% but not lower. This is due to methaemoglobin absorbing light strongly at both 940 nm, where the absorbance of oxyHb is slightly more than deoxyHb and at 640 nm where the absorbance of deoxyHb in red light is more than oxyHb. The pulse oximeter works out the ratio of absorbed light at these two wavelengths. When the ratio equals unity there is an oximeter reading of 85%. Hence a patient may be grossly hypoxaemic with methaemoglobinaemia but the pulse oximeter will read 85% and not less.[27]

- The pulse oximeter signal is one way of monitoring brachial artery compression during shoulder arthroscopy but will not exclude traction or pressure injury to nerves which will often precede arterial compression.[28]

> A sudden reduction in pulse oximeter reading maybe due to
>
> apnoea or reduced tidal volume;
>
> reduced inspired oxygen;
>
> increased oxygen consumption – hyperpyrexia, thyroid crisis;
>
> reduced cardiac output.

Pulmonary Artery Catheters
(Figure 41)

Use: Measurement of cardiovascular parameters and to guide the effectiveness of therapy.

- Pulmonary oedema. Pulmonary capillary wedge pressure:
  High in – cardiac failure, fluid overload.
  Normal/low in – increased pulmonary membrane permeability.

- Fluid therapy. Cardiac output and vascular resistance to assess fluid therapy.

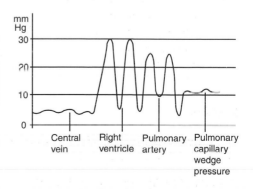

Figure 41 – Pulmonary artery catheter trace.

- Shock management. Differentiate:
  Cardiogenic – inotrope, vasodilator.
  Septic – fluid, vasopressor, inotrope.
  Hypovoaemia – fluid.

Treatment	Parameters	Conditions
Fluid	Low cardiac output, low vascular resistance	Hypovolaemic states
Inotrope	Low cardiac output, high pulmonary capillary wedge pressure	Poor cardiac function
Vasopressor	Low systemic vascular resistance	Relative hypovolaemia, anaphylaxis
Vasodilator	Low cardiac output, high systemic vascular resistance with normal cardiac output	Poor cardiac function

Cardiac output curves

- Normal – rapid ascent and return to base line in 10–15 s.

- High output – short duration curve, no tail.

- Low output – rapid ascent but a long tail with slow return to baseline.

- Tricuspid incompetence – slow rise and long tail.

Check catheter before use,

(a) transducer and monitor calibration,
(b) balloon inflation and inspection,
(c) thermistor test, (d) proximal and distal lumen attachment to transducer, (e) fluid flush.

Check for damping by coiling the catheter in one hand and shaking up and down. The oscilloscope should show high spike waves from both lumen. Now flick the catheter and a clear spike shows that the system is free of air bubbles.[29]

- This shake-flick test is recommended to test for pressure wave damping due to air bubbles within the lumens. In order to ensure that only the distal port trace is observed while advancing the catheter the test is performed with the thumb of one hand occluding the proximal port of the catheter while the catheter is held coiled in the same hand. The proximal port trace should then change from a continuous low–pressure horizontal line to a continuous high–pressure horizontal line, while the distal port trace should be a high spiking waveform.[30]

Obtaining a wedge pressure

- Monitor ECG for: dysrhythmias of atrium and ventricle on passing catheter. No treatment is usually required other than to stop and reposition the catheter.

- Check the wedge is complete by watching a fall in pressure when the balloon is inflated. Better to check the waveform mirrors the left atrial contraction by linking with the P of the ECG and not the T wave. If in doubt deflate balloon and withdraw catheter and then repeat.

Catheter knot

- A true knot in a thermal dilution catheter is rare compared to the presence of a loop. Even less frequently the knot tightens with gentle pulling. To remove a knotted catheter the proximal end of the Swan–Ganz catheter is cut. The 8 Fr catheter introducer sheath is removed and replaced by a larger 10 Fr sheath. The knot is now pulled into the sheath and the whole removed with minimum vein damage.[31]

References

1. Guidelines for the Use of Non-steroidal Anti-inflammatory Drugs in the Perioperative Period. Royal College of Anaesthetists, London, March 1998.
2. Edwards RB. Paediatric pain chart. *Anaesthesia* 1994; **49:** 91–2.
3. White JB, Stow P. Rationale and experience with visual analogue toys. *Anaesthesia* 1985; **40:** 601–3.
4. Cross GD. Simple device for the assessment of local anaesthetic blocks in children. *Anaesthesia* 1987; **42:** 84.
5. Harrison GR, Worsley MH, Clark C. Inhaled opiates. *Anaesthesia* 1990; **45:** 992.
6. Worsley MH, Macleod AD, Brodie MJ, Asbury AJ, Clark C. Inhaled fentanyl as a method of analgesia. *Anaesthesia* 1990; **45:** 449–51.
7. Cassuto J et al. Inhibition of postoperative pain by continuous low-dose intravenous infusion of lidocaine. *Anesthesia and Analgesia* 1985; **64:** 971–4.
8. Haynes TK et al. Intra-articular morphine and bupivacaine analgesia after arthroscopic knee surgery. *Anaesthesia* 1994; **49:** 54–6.
9. Bull PT, Mowbray MJ, Markham SJ. Subcutaneous opioids: the painless approach. *Anaesthesia* 1992; **47:** 276.
10. Ahuja S, Datta A, Krishna A, Bhattacharya A. Infra-orbital nerve block for pain relief of postoperative pain following cleft lip surgery in infants. *Anaesthesia* 1994; **49:** 441–4.
11. Knox DJ, McLeod BJ, Goucke CR. Acute phantom limb pain controlled by ketamine. *Anaesthesia and Intensive Care* 1995; **23:** 620–2.
12. Sellers WFS. A test for reflex response. *Anaesthesia* 1981; **36:** 538.
13. O'Donovan N, Healy TEJ, Faragher EB, Wilkins RG, Hamilton AA. Postoperative backache: the use of an inflatable wedge. *British Journal of Anaesthesia* 1986; **58:** 280–3.
14. Snyder AR, Ilko R. Topical nitroglycerin for intraoperative penile turgescence. *Anesthesia and Analgesia* 1987; **66:** 1022–3.
15. MacNaman, Rijat MS, Quinton DN. The changing profile of poisoning and its management. *Journal of the Royal College of Medicine* 1996; **89:** 608–10.
16. Hall AP. Ecstasy and the anaesthetists. *British Journal of Anaestehsia* 1997; **79:** 697–8.
17. Jones NC, Ginsburg R. Problems due to substance abuse. *Anaesthesia Review* 1997; **14:** 243–71.
18. Shanon M. Toxicology reviews. *Pediatric Emergency Care* 1998; **14:** 293–8.
19. Doyle E, Best C. Whole bowel irrigation in acute poisoning. *British Journal of Anaesthesia* 1993; **71:** 464.
20. James MFM , Hift RJ. Porphyrias. *British Journal of Anaesthesia* 2000; **85:** 143–53.
21. Prasad MK, Puri GD, Chari P. Glove finger for fixing pulse oximeter. *Anaesthesia* 1994; **49:** 831.
22. Bardoczky GI, Engelman E, d'Hollander AA. One more use of a Vinyl glove: ready made protection for the reusable pulse oximeter monitoring probe. *Anesthesiology* 1989; **71:** 999.
23. Ackerman WE, Juneja MM, Baumann RC, Kaczorowski DM. The use of vinyl glove does not effect pulse oximeter monitoring. *Anesthesiology* 1989; **70:** 558–9.
24. Gupta A, Vegfors M. A simple solution. *Anaesthesia* 1992; **47:** 822.
25. Brooks TD, Paulus DA, Winkle WE. Infrared heat lamps interfere with pulse oximeters. *Anesthesiology* 1984; **61:** 630.
26. Ransing Th, Rosenberg J. Pulse oximetry in severe anaemia. *Intensive Care Medicine* 1992; **18:** 125–6.
27. Delwood L et al. Methaemoglobin and pulse oximetry. *Anaesthesia* 1992; **47:** 80.
28. Gibbs N, Handel J. Pulse oximetry during shoulder arthroscopy. *Anesthesiology* 1987; **67:** 150–1.
29. Mihm FG, Ashton JPA. Pulmonary artery catheters – the shake-flick test. *Anesthesiology* 1983; **59:** 262–3.
30. DiNardo JA, Satwicz PR. Occlusion-shake test for pulmonary artery catheters. *Anesthesiology* 1984; **61:** 349–50.
31. Castella M. True knot in a Swan–Ganz catheter on a central venous catheter: a simple trick for percutaneous removal. *Intensive Care Medicine* 1996; **22:** 830–1.

Rate–Pressure Product (RPP)

RPP is the multiple of heart rate and systolic blood pressure. A value over 12,000 during anaesthesia is an indicator of increased sympathetic activity. This may be due to

- awareness,

- hypoxia,

- pain,

- hypovolaemia,

- hypercarbia,

- catecholamine – endogenous or exogenous.

A patient with ischaemic heart disease will complain of anginal pain at a RPP of 20,000. Patients undergoing coronary bypass surgery show ECG ischaemia at 12,000. Control of RPP with beta blockade and vasodilatation is recommended to reduce perioperative myocardial ischaemia.[1]

Ring Removal

- Rings can be removed from a finger by lubrication of the finger with soap or oil.

- A string is twisted several times around the finger, starting at the tip and working

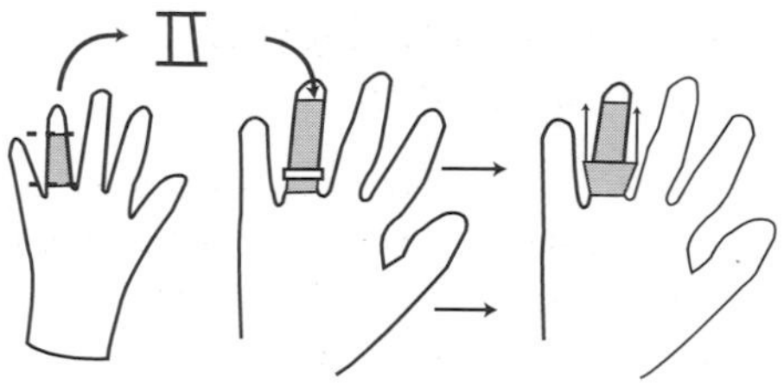

Figure 42 – Use of rubber glove finger to remove ring.

downwards so that the proximal end passes under the ring. The distal end is now tightened to ease the ring up and off.

- The finger part of a rubber surgical glove is cut off and slipped over the finger and under the ring. The segment beyond the ring is turned inside out and pulled towards the finger tip with a twisting motion. This technique can be used when the finger is burnt or otherwise traumatised[2] (Figure 42).

- As a last resort a ring may have to be cut off.

References

1. Jones RM, Knight PR, Hill AB. Rate pressure product. *Anaesthesia* 1980; **35:** 1010–11.
2. Shimizu R. Another simple method for ring removal. *Anesthesiology* 1995; **83:** 1133–4.

Scavenging the T-piece Breathing Circuit

A number of suggestions exist for scavenging the Jackson Rees modification of the Ayre's T-piece breathing circuit. Many involve connecting the tail of reservoir bag to suction. There must be a venting system to prevent direct suction on the bag.

- The coaxial plastic connection is cut from the patient end of the Bain system. The central tube is left attached for 2–3 cm and a long connector is used to link the central lumen into the tail of the reservoir bag. It should be pushed well in to prevent kinking. A scavenging connection is attached to the outer part on the other side of the connector. This allows entrainment of air when no gas comes out of the tail of the bag.

- The nozzle of a bladder syringe is inserted into the tail end of paediatric reservoir bag. Holes are made in the nozzle and syringe barrel. The scavenging system is fitted over the barrel, held with tape if needed.[1]

- A small reservoir bag can be used in place of the syringe, connected between its tail and the tail of the bag on the T piece. The main problem is twisting at the connection.[2]

Bag in bag

- The reservoir bag is placed inside a larger transparent bag, which is attached to a scavenging hose.[3]

Others

- There are several descriptions using two interconnected T pieces.[4–6]

- A scavenging dish is fitted at the head end of the operating table in such a way that the gas escaping from the open tail of the reservoir bag of the T piece empties into the dish.[7,8]

Scores of Illness

There are a number of scoring systems, some are simple and others complex. They attempt, with varying degrees of success, to predict outcome.

ASA

Score: 1. normal, 2. disease that is controlled and does not affect life, 3. disease with a small limit in function, 4. severe disease which is a threat to life and limits function, 5. moribund patient not expected to live past 24 h.

The ASA score assesses the chronic medical state of the patient. It makes no assessment of operative risk, the current medical condition or any anaesthetic difficulties. A graded anaesthetic score is suggested to use along side the ASA score.[9]

The patient could be scored along the following lines:

1. No additional risk.

2. Minor factors. Dental work, URTI, pseudocholinesterase abnormalities.

3. Major factors. Malignant hyperthermia susceptibility, moderate physiological disturbance following trauma, sepsis, head injury, pre-eclampsia.

4. Life threatening factors. Acute airway obstruction, eclampsia, severe physiological disturbance following trauma, sepsis, morbid obesity.

Scores of illness[10] include:

- Acute physiological and chronic health evaluation (APACHE),[11] trauma score (TS) combined with injury severity score (ISS) to make trauma and revised injury severity score (TRISS).[12] These scores do not assess outcome or morbidity nor do they take into account the culture and motivation of the patient. Other assessments include cardiac risk index[13] (Goldman cardiac risk index) and Glasgow coma scale (GCS, as below).[14]

- A simple system based on clinical observation provides an objective measure of illness for critically ill patients in Africa. A high score is a good predictor of poor outcome. The clinical sickness score (CSS, as below) records pulse rate, blood pressure respiratory rate, urine output, GCS, temperature and age. Each item is given a rating from 0 to +4.[15]

- A co-morbidity score of smoking habit, alcohol intake, non-cured malignancy, treated diabetes mellitus, splenectomy, previous major surgery or antibiotics within 2 months of admission, cardiogenic shock or CPR is claimed to show a high correlation with death rate in septicaemia and with more sophisticated scores such as APACHE.[16]

Stethoscope

- The use of a precordial stethoscope placed over the left thorax in infants allows for the instant monitoring of respiration and heart sounds from before induction of anaesthesia until the recovery period. It is more versatile than the oesophageal stethoscope. The stethoscope bell can be attached to rubber tubing and a microphone fitted onto the tubing. The sounds can be amplified, played over a tape recorder system and heard 3–4 m away.[17]

- Place a stethoscope over the left precordium to monitor for heart rate, respiration with left lung air entry.

- Use if there is a risk of air embolism as an alternative to a Doppler.

- To enable the listener to monitor both sides of the chest at the same time a double head stethoscope is made by joining the flexible

Glasgow coma scale (GCS)

Score	Eyes	Verbal response	Motor response
1	Shut	None	None
2	Open to pain	Noises	Extension (brainstem lesion)
3	Open to command	Confused words	Abnormal flexion
4	Spontaneously open	Confused sentences	Withdrawal to pain
5		Orientated	Localises to pain
6			Moves to command

Clinical sickness score (CSS)

Score	4	3	2	1	0	1	2	3	4
Pulse	>180	140–179	110–139		70–109		55–69	40–54	<40
Systolic BP	>200	170–199	150–169	140–149	100–139	80–99	60–79		<60
Respiratory rate	>50	35–49		25–34	12–24	10–11	6–9		IPPV
Urine volume	Anuria		<50 ml/h		50–100 ml/h		>200 ml/h		
Temperature (°C)	>40	39			38	36–37	33–35	31–32	30	29
GCS*	Subtract from 15								
Age (years)	61+			51–60	41–50	<40			

*Glasgow coma scale: *Intensive Care Medicine* 1989; **15**: 467–70.

tubing from each ear piece to separate diaphragms.A diaphragm is strapped over each side of the chest wall.[18–20]

Oesophageal sounds

During anaesthesia the sounds from the oesophageal stethoscope can change if it is in the lower half of the oesophagus. Muffling of the heart and breath sounds, sometimes accompanied by swallowing noises, is usually a sign that the patient is becoming light.[21]

The change in sounds is related to the non-striated musculature in the lower half of the oesophagus, which is not affected by muscle relaxants except curare. There is a progressive increase in lower oesophageal contractility during lightening of anaesthesia[22]

Suction

- A negative pressure of −60 kPa is created by hospital piped suction. This will damage mucosa and rapidly withdraw air from the lungs. Suction should be applied for the minimum time possible.

- Tracheal suction: preoxygenate with 100% oxygen for 3 min. Pass the catheter into the trachea without suction. Apply suction while withdrawing the catheter. Re-expand the lung with 100% oxygen.If there are more secretions repeat the whole procedure, but do not continue to suck for longer than it takes to withdraw the catheter.

References

1. Hasselt G van, Phillips J. T-piece scavenging: simple alternatives. *Anaesthesia* 1994; **49**: 263–4.
2. Chan MSH. A new T-piece scavenging system. *Anaesthesia and Intensive Care* 1993; **21**: 899.
3. Chan MSH, Kong AS. T piece scavenging – the double-bag system. *Anaesthesia* 1993; **48**: 647.
4. Barake A, Muallem M. Scavenging of anaesthesia gases using the double T-piece system. *Anaesthesia* 1978; **50**: 974.
5. Baraka A, Muallem M. Scavenging by the double T-piece circuit. *Anaesthesia* 1993; **48**: 1116.
6. Kumar CM. Another antipollution device for the Jackson-Rees modification of Ayre's T-piece. *Anaesthesia* 1991; **46**: 792.
7. Hatch DJ, Miles R, Wagstaff M. Anaesthetic scavenging system for paediatric and adult use. *Anaesthesia* 1980; **35**: 496–9.
8. Sik MJ, Lewis RB, Eveleigh DJ. Assessment of a scavenging device for use in paediatric anaesthesia. *British Journal of Anaesthesia* 1990; **64**: 117–23.
9. Lake A, Williams EGN. ASA classification and perioperative variables: graded anaesthesia score? *British Journal of Anaesthesia* 1997; **78**: 229.
10. Ridley S. Severity of illness scoring systems and performance appraisal. *Anaesthesia* 1998; **53**: 1185–94.
11. Knaus WA, Draper EA, Wagenr DP, Zimmerman JE. APACHE 11: a severity of disease classification system. *Critical Care Medicine* 1985; **13**: 818–29.
12. Boyd CR, Tolson MA, Copes WS. Evaluating trauma care: the TRISS method. Trauma score and the injury score. *Journal of Trauma* 1987; **27**: 370–8.
13. Goldman LB, Caldera DL, Nussbaum SR. *New England Journal of Medicine* 1977; **297**: 845–50.
14. Teasdale G, Jennett B. *Lancet* 1974; **ii**: 81–3.
15. Watters DAK, Wilson IH, Sinclair JR, Ngandu N. A clinical sickness score for the critically ill in central Africa. *Intensive Care Medicine* 1989; **15**: 467–70.
16. Pittet D, Thievent B, Wenzel RP, Gurman G, Suter PM. Importance of pre-existing co-morbidities for prognosis of septicaemia in critically ill patients. *Intensive Care Medicine* 1993; **19**: 265–72.
17. Ginott N. Vacuum stethoscope attached to a tape recorder. *Anaesthesia* 1977; **32**: 896–7.
18. Walker JA, Mathur AK. A bilateral stethoscope. *Anaesthesia* 1983; **38**: 164.
19. Lee E. Of stethoscopes and stopcocks. *Anaesthesia and Analgesia* 1991; **73**: 99.
20. Brill SL. A two head stethoscope. *Anesthesia and Analgesia* 1996; **82**: 887.
21. Meyer RM. Esophageal stethoscope can reveal light anaesthesia. *Anesthesia and Analgesia* 1986; **65**: 319.
22. Evans J. Esophageal activity and light anaesthesia. *Anesthesia and Analgesia* 1987; **66**: 196–7.

Throat Spray

Individual sprays should be used to prevent cross contamination. The cannula can pick up material on the outside. A negative pressure on the inside will suck fluid into the lumen.

Options

- Use an individual cannula for each patient.

- A 14G intravenous cannula used as a sheath over the existing attachment.[1]

- Specific doses placed in individual applicators by the pharmacy. This limits the total dose available in a situation where overdose is likely.

Transfer

A large sheet under the patient is used for a sliding transfer. The sheet will usually be plastic but in difficult circumstances plastic bin bags can be used either to slide on the bag or it will roll by cutting off the end, like a caterpillar tread on a tank.[2]

Transfer of head injury patients[3]

Patients should be stable before transfer.

1. Airway: usually intubated if GCS < 9.

2. Respiration: arterial oxygen > 13 kPa, arterial carbon dioxide 4.0–4.5 kPa, or normocapnoea 5.6 kPa, paralysed and ventilated.
   Cerebral blood flow (CBF) = 59 ml/100 mg/min. CBF is proportional to P_aCO_2 when mean arterial pressure (MAP) is 20–80 mmHg. Cerebral use

of oxygen is 3.5 ml/100 mg/min, 50 ml or 20% of body's oxygen requirement, 250 ml.

3. Circulation: systolic pressure > 120 mmHg, pulse < 100/min.

4. Good venous access.

5. Assess head injury: GCS stable not changing.

6. Assess all other injuries: neck, chest, abdomen, pelvis and long bones; need for blood/fluids during transfer.

7. Monitor: ECG, pulse oximeter, BP, capnography and ventilation parameters.

8. Support equipment and staff should be available in the ambulance and at the sending and receiving hospitals during transfer.

9. If the patient is not expected to survive the journey they should not set out.

10. A transfer checklist should be completed including trained staff, patient's notes and X-rays, whereabouts of going, drugs and fluids, monitors, suction, money for breakdown and tolls, portable phone.

References

1. Nott MR. An alternative throat spray. *Anaesthesia* 1991; **46:** 518.
2. Yamashita M, Matsuki A. Use of a garbage bag for patient transfer. *Anesthesiology* 1983; **59:** 168.
3. Recommendations for the transfer of patients with acute head injuries to neurosurgical units. The Association of Anaesthetists of Great Britain and Ireland, December 1996.

Veins

The dorsum of the hand is often chosen for venous access as the veins are superficial. The assistant should apply gentle pressure to the forearm, sufficient to prevent venous flow out of the arm, but not so much that arterial blood is prevented from entering the hand. Gentle proximal traction helps to straighten the vein. A small intradermal bleb of lidocaine rapidly anaesthetises the skin before cannulation.

The forearm, using the cephalic vein at the base of the thumb or branches of the basilic vein in the medial forearm is a better site for fixing an intravenous infusion. No part of the infusion should be fixed across a joint to prevent displacement on movement.

Difficult veins

Look everywhere before starting. There may be a better vein on the dorsum of the foot, dorsal surface of the forearm on the ulnar side, neck or forehead – the temporal artery and vein can be difficult to differentiate in children.

Think of an interosseous needle.

Hand veins can be encouraged to vasodilate by

- enclosure in a pair of surgical gloves;[1]

- wrapping with aluminium foil;[2]

- applying glyceryl trinitrate ointment to a small area on the dorsum of the hand. This increases the visibility of the veins for cannulation. Some patients may complain of headache and excess ointment should be removed after cannulation;[3]

- two fibre-optic lights, 3–4 cm apart illuminate non-visible veins without thermal injury. The most reliable areas are the forearm, dorsum of hand and volar surface of the wrist. Velcro straps can be used to hold the lights in place.[4] Such a light source is found on rigid oesophagoscopes.

A small bore cannula used as a guide for a larger bore cannula.

To force the distension of peripheral veins:

- A small cannula is introduced. A tourniquet at 50–60 mmHg is applied to the distal limb. Crystalloid is infused through the small bore cannula; 0.5 ml of methylene blue added to 500 ml of crystalloid, or compatible blood makes the veins more visible and warm fluid is more effective than cold fluid.[5]

- Enter vein with cannula and use a Seldinger technique to insert a guide wire through the small cannula; withdraw the cannula then a large bore cannula is passed over the guide wire.[6]

To detect that a cannula is in a vein:

Once a cannula is in place a palpating hand proximal to the site of insertion will detect a thrill when a few ml of saline is injected. Auscultation over the vein proximal to the tip of the catheter will hear a bruit on injection. No thrill or bruit suggest extravascular placement.[7]

Central venous catheters

The central veins can be cannulated from the basilic, axillary, subclavian, jugular and femoral vein in children.

Planes used to describe needle direction. The sagittal plane is in line with the sagittal cranial suture. A plane as if the body is cut from front to back along a line drawn from the nose to the umbilicus. The coronal plane is a line as if the front of the body is separated from the back of the body along the mid-axillary line.

Indications for central venous catheterisation: monitor right atrial pressure which indicates preload, right ventricular end diastolic pressure (RVEDP), access when other veins are not accessible, Swan–Ganz catheter for pressure values and calculations of cardiac output and vascular resistance.

Contraindications: sepsis, clotting defect, unskilled.

Internal jugular vein

> Position: supine with head turned to opposite side, 15–30° head down to distend vein and prevent air embolism. Use aseptic technique and infiltrate with LA before using a large cannula.
>
> Consider a superficial cervical plexus block by placing 2–5 ml LA at the mid-point of the posterior border of sternomastoid.

Vein runs from deep to mastoid process to sternoclavicular joint. The vein is approached at the apex of the anterior triangle to avoid a pneumothorax. A needle is inserted in the angle between the sternal and clavicular heads of sternomastoid 4–7 cm above the clavicle.

The carotid artery is retracted medially and the needle is inserted at 30–40° to the skin (coronal plane) directed to the ipsilateral nipple. A give is felt as the fascia of the carotid sheath is penetrated and then the vein. Aspirate for blood. The needle is inserted a further 1 cm before a wire is passed, then a dilator and then the catheter.

Ultrasound guidance of the needle insertion is recommended to reduce the incidence of complications for all internal jugular cannulations.

Other approaches to the vein

The neck is extended to 10°. A transverse line is drawn halfway between the cricoid and thyroid cartilages. The pads of the middle three fingers are placed on the lateral aspect of the larynx with the tips pointing posteriorly, along the line of the carotid artery. Immediately lateral to the fingers on the marked line local anaesthetic is infiltrated and a seeker needle is inserted. The needle is directed parallel to the sagittal plane and 30–40° to the coronal plane. The needle is redirected more laterally until the vein is cannulated.[8]

High approach

- A high approach to the vein uses the carotid triangle bounded by sternomastoid laterally, posterior belly of digastric and hyoideus. The vein is superficial in this position. A pneumothorax is less likely and catheter fixation is easier. The head is turned to the opposite side, the carotid artery palpated and a point lateral to the artery as high as possible below the mandible chosen for the point of skin puncture. After infiltration of local anaesthetic a seeking needle is passed caudally at 75–85° to the coronal plane[9] (Figures 43 and 44).

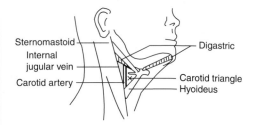

Figure 43 – High approach to internal jugular vein.

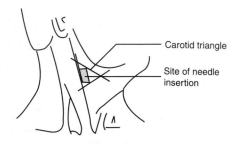

Figure 44 – Site of needle insertion.

Neutral head position

- Patients with a cervical injury who require venous access should keep the head in a neutral position. Subclavian or femoral veins are alternatives. The head is neutral, the needle is introduced at a point lateral to the cricoid cartilage and on a line drawn cephalad from the lateral insertion of the clavicular head of sternomastoid on the clavicle. The clavicular insertion is easily identified as a palpating finger rolls off the muscle into an indentation, above the clavicle, at this level[10] (Figure 45).

- Another neutral position technique uses only the carotid artery as a landmark and has the advantage of being independent of other physical variants. The patient is tilted slightly head down to distend the internal jugular vein. The head is not rotated. The course, depth and lateral wall of the carotid artery are identified. The needle is introduced at the level of the prominence of the thyroid cartilage, 0.5 cm lateral to the carotid artery, at 30–45° to the skin (coronal plane). The initial puncture is made close to the artery and if unsuccessful subsequent attempts are made with the needle directed more laterally.[11]

In difficult cases: 22G spinal needle as an guide.

- To reduce haematoma formation a 22G 150 mm spinal needle with the stylet removed and a syringe attached, is passed through the lumen of a 16G or 14G 100 mm cannula. The leading 40 mm portion of the 22G needle is used to locate the vein. Once a flush back is obtained the cannula is passed over it as if the 22G needle were a guide wire. The needle is advanced about 6 cm into the vein.[12,13]

- The patient is placed supine and slightly head down with the head turned to the opposite side. A 22G 100 mm spinal needle, with syringe attached, is advanced parallel to the trachea and lateral to the carotid artery at a 30–45° angle to the skin until it enters the vein. A 14G needle is now advanced behind and parallel to the spinal needle. The spinal needle is now withdrawn.[14]

The obese

Bony landmarks can be used when other landmarks are lost as in obese patients. The

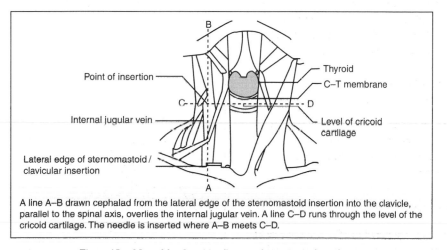

A line A–B drawn cephalad from the lateral edge of the sternomastoid insertion into the clavicle, parallel to the spinal axis, overlies the internal jugular vein. A line C–D runs through the level of the cricoid cartilage. The needle is inserted where A–B meets C–D.

Figure 45 – Neutral head position for cannulating internal jugular vein.

puncture site is the intersection of a line on the axial plane at the level of the cricoid cartilage and a line from the mastoid process to the sternal end of clavicle. The carotid artery is palpated just medial to the puncture site. The needle is introduced toward the clavicular notch, in the clavicle, at an angle of 30–45° with the coronal plane. The clavicular notch is about 1 cm lateral to the sternal end of the clavicle[15] (Figure 46).

Children

A posterior approach for cannulating the internal jugular vein is described for use in children. Placing a support – rolled towel or fluid bag – behind the shoulders and the head rotated to the contralateral side extends the neck. A small incision is made in the skin half to two-thirds of the way along the lateral border of sternomastoid coming up from the clavicle, after infiltrating the skin with local anaesthetic. A needle is inserted and advanced towards a point just beneath the ipsilateral sternoclavicular joint with continuous aspiration. The needle should not be advanced beyond the clavicle. The angle is changed slightly if the vein is not found in the first attempt[16] (Figure 47).

Subclavian vein

Position: supine, slight head down tilt. Arm to side and a bag between shoulder blades if groove between deltoid and pectoralis is deep. Start with the left side to avoid the thoracic duct.

Needle entry 1.5–2 cm below clavicle at mid-point or slightly lateral, confirmed by palpating subclavian artery above mid-point of clavicle. Direct needle to mid-point of clavicle on opposite side, over first rib and under clavicle. If the subclavian artery, which lies posteriorly and above the vein, is

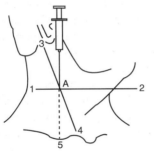

A – Needle entry site for internal jugular vein puncture at intersection of

line 1–2: axial plane at cricoid level
line 3–4: between mastoid process and sternal end of clavicle
Needle aimed at 5 – notch of clavicle

Figure 46 – Landmark in obese patient.

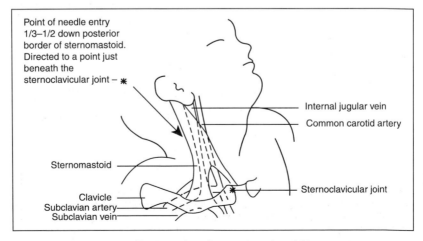

Figure 47 – Internal jugular vein approach in children.

punctured apply pressure and redirect the needle anteriorly and inferiorly.

Infraclavicular approach to the axillary vein

The infraclavicular approach to axillary vein is safer than approaches to the internal jugular vein from the neck. The structures most likely to be damaged are superior to the vein therefore the needle is aimed "low". The needle should not be advanced beneath the clavicle. This is not an easy technique but there is a low incidence of complications, the most common being arterial puncture.

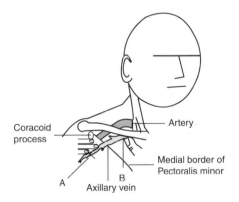

Coracoid process

Artery

Medial border of Pectoralis minor

A   B
    Axillary vein

Figure 48 – Infra-clavicular approach to axillary vein.

Finding the axillary vein:

1. The axillary vein is the continuation of the basilic vein extending from the lower border of teres major to the outer border of the first rib. The patient is supine, with 15° head down tilt. The arm is abducted to 45° making the vein straight from basilic to subclavian vein (Figures 48 and 49).

A mark is made on the skin three fingers (5 cm) below the coracoid process, a second mark is made in the grove below the medial end of the clavicle where the thorax just becomes palpable. These two marks are joined and a third point marked where the line crosses the medial border of pectoralis minor. The needle is introduced on the line and lateral to the medial border of pectoralis minor. It is passed medially aiming to enter the vein medial to the pectoralis minor. Use a small gauge seeking needle to avoid a haematoma due to puncturing the axillary artery.[17]

2. Two points, point A, three fingers width or 5 cm below the lower margin of the coracoid, and point B, at the junction of the medial one-fourth and lateral

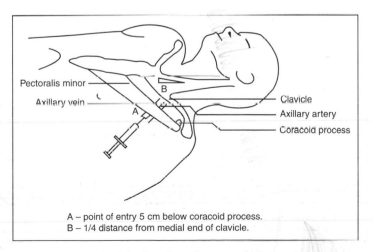

Pectoralis minor

Axillary vein

B

A

Clavicle

Axillary artery

Coracoid process

A – point of entry 5 cm below coracoid process.
B – 1/4 distance from medial end of clavicle.

Figure 49 – Infra-clavicular axillary vein cannulation.

three-fourths of the clavicle, are marked. The needle enters at A directed towards B. It will pierce the pectoralis minor muscle before entering the axillary vein[18] (Figure 49).

3. Consider an inverted three-sided pyramid between the suprasternal notch, the acromioclavicular joint and a point equidistant along the margin of pectoralis major. The axillary vein is cannulated at the apex of the pyramid.[19]

External jugular vein

The use of a J wire passed through a 18G or 20G, 38 mm overneedle teflon catheter, inserted into the external jugular vein is an alternative access to the central veins.[20]

The external jugular vein can be distended, even in the sitting position, by placing a stethoscope about the neck to act as a tourniquet.[21]

Differentiating venous from arterial cannulation

- The colour of the blood is not a reliable differentiation.

- Transducer for venous or arterial waveform.

- Arterial gas analysis.[22]

Tunnelling

To avoid cutting the catheter while tunnelling:

- The introducing needle is tunnelled from the proximal side and the cannula cut across to take the catheter.[23]

- Insert only the needle outwards from the site of the original incision. The cannula is now threaded over the needle from the other end and the needle withdrawn. The catheter is now threaded

down the cannula without risk of damage.[24]

- Consider using Steristip wound closures. These will remove the risk of cutting the catheter with the needle of a suture and infection is less likely to be introduced near the catheter.[25]

Alternative sites for large bore cannulae

Basilic vein

- Situated in the antecubital fossa medial to the biceps muscle tendon and superficial to the brachial artery.

- One technique involves the use of a 14G needle and cannula. The basilic vein, on the medial side of the antecubital fossa is chosen over the cephalic as the former makes a direct line into the axillary vein. The arm is cleaned and draped and the 14G cannula is used as an introducer for a 16G 60 cm catheter or an introducer wire.[26]

Advantages

- Easily accessible for short cannulae or using a Seldinger technique for advancing a longer catheter from the axillary vein into the superior vena cava.

- No pneumothorax, haematoma easily controlled by pressure.

Disadvantages

- Thrombophlebitis.

- Difficult to fix cannula and maintain patient comfort.

- Possible arterial cannulation.

Femoral vein

Medial to femoral artery below inguinal ligament.

Advantages

- Easy to palpate artery and make cannulation with thigh extended. Used in small children.
- Seldinger technique for introducing catheter into the inferior vena cava.

Disadvantages

- Trauma to femoral artery or nerve.
- Difficult to fix catheter and keep site clean.

Central venous pressure (CVP)

- Starling described the relationship between cardiac muscle fibre length and the force of contraction. These parameters can be indirectly assessed from the central venous pressure representing the fibre length and the cardiac output or blood pressure representing the force of contraction. The relationship between these two measurements under different clinical situations are well illustrated in the graphs[27,28] (Figure 50).

- A fluid challenge (Figure 51) can be used to differentiate between normovolaemia, hypovolaemia and heart failure. If the CVP is 0–5 cmH$_2$O rapidly infuse 500–1000 ml crystalloid. In normovolaemia the pressure will rise and return to a baseline within 20 min. In hypovolaemia the rise is less and the return to baseline is quicker. In heart failure the pressure does not return to the baseline. If the CVP is already high the test should be repeated but using a smaller volume of crystalloid of 200–500 ml.

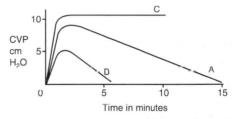
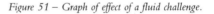

A – Normal B Hypovolaemic C – Heart failure/overload

Figure 51 – Graph of effect of a fluid challenge.

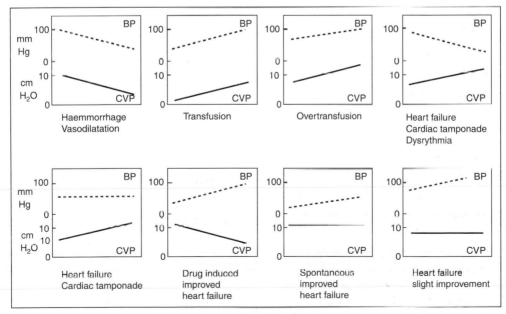

Figure 50 – Relationship of BP and CVP.

141

Measuring CVP

Clinically

Observe the height of the filling in the neck veins with the patient sitting at 40° to the horizontal. A rise in height can be due to valves in these veins, heart failure, increased preload and obstruction to venous flow in the mediastinum. Or observe the veins on the hand and then raise the arm until these veins collapse. Measure the vertical distance from the hand to the right atrium.

Position for catheter tip (Figure 52)

Clinically: The patient is supine. With the introducer on the chest wall the catheter is judged to be at the level, or slightly below the sternal angle. The sternal angle level is above the junction of the SVC and the right atrium. This can leave the catheter high in the SVC or in the left innominate vein if coming from the left.

Chest X-ray

- Position the catheter tip at the level of the carina on X-ray.

- A chest x-ray taken in deep inspiration will show the carina at the level of T6. The trachea elongates in inspiration. In expiration the carina will be at T4/5.

- The SVC is 6 cm long. The carina is 3.5 cm higher than the SVC/atrial junction.

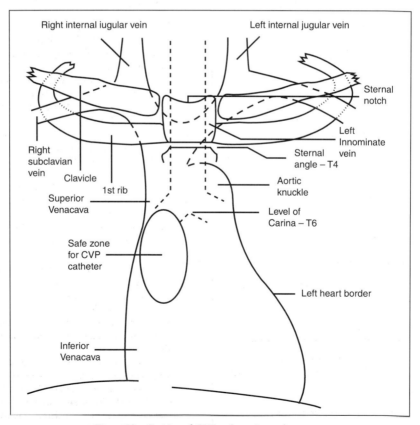

Figure 52 – Position of CVP catheter tip on chest x-ray.

- The sternal angle is usually higher at T4. Placing the catheter tip above the carina level increases the risk of thrombosis, and perforation if coming from the left.

Fixing the zero for a CVP manometer

- Take a length of tubing such as suction tubing. Fill it half-full with coloured water and then join the ends together to make a continuous tube. One fluid level is placed on the supine patient at the mid-axillary line or sternal notch. The other fluid level is placed along side the manometer column to give the zero level.[29]

- A half-filled 500 ml bag of saline, to which dye has been added, is attached to about 2 m of wide bore tubing. The bag is placed on the sternum and the tubing fixed vertically to give a fluid level.[30] This zero will move if the patient is moved.

A transducer should always be level with the right atrium and move with the patient.

Ventilator Pressure

If inflation pressure increases or drops consider problems with

- machine,

- airway and tube,

- patient's lung.

Increased inflation pressure consider:

Machine. Disconnect and use a self-inflating bag and one-way valve.

Tube. Exclude oesophageal intubation, measure expired carbon dioxide. Consider passing a bougie, which should stop at 40 cm, deflate cuff, and remove tube over an introducer.

Patient. Pneumothorax, bronchospasm, pulmonary oedema, aspiration.

Give oxygen and specific treatment.

When the compliances of two lungs are different two ventilators may be needed to control oxygenation without increasing the volume or pressure in one lung at the expense of the other. Synchronising the ventilators is a problem.

One ventilator can be used with two sets of ventilator tubing, one fitted with a clamp constrictor. A double lumen tube is used to prevent soiling from one tube to the other. This arrangement may be useful following chest injury with haemoptysis, particularly if both lungs are damaged,[31] or a bronchopleural fistula with air leak from one lung.

References

1. Kalmanovitch DVA. Dilatation of hand veins. *Anaesthesia* 1991; **46:** 517.
2. McLaren P. Dilating peripheral veins. *Anaesthesia and Intensive Care* 1994; **22:** 318.
3. Parakh SC, Patwari A. Experience with 2% nitroglycerine ointment as an aid to venepuncture. *British Journal of Anaesthesia* 1986; **58:** 822.
4. Dinner M. Transillumination to facilitate venipuncture in children. *Anesthesia and Analgesia* 1992; **74:** 467.
5. McCrory J. Facilitation of wide bore cannula insertion. *Anaesthesia* 1988; **43:** 612.
6. Turtle M. Multiple use of a single vein. *Anaesthesia* 1985; **40:** 1243.
7. Dean VS. Additional test to confirm placement of paediatric lines. *Anesthesia and Analgesia* 1996; **82:** 1113.
8. Latto IP, Hughes JA, Falconer RJ. An assessment of an alternative method of internal jugular vein cannulation. *Anaesthesia* 1992; **47:** 1047–50.
9. Messahael FM, Al-Mazroa AA. Cannulation of the internal jugular vein. *Anaesthesia* 1992; **47:** 842–4.
10. Willeford KL, Reitan JA. Neutral position for placement of internal jugular vein catheters. *Anaesthesia* 1994; **49:** 203–4.
11. Oda M et al. The para-carotid approach for internal jugular vein catheterisation. *Anaesthesia* 1981; **36:** 896–900.

12. Christian CM. Cannulation of the internal jugular vein: variation on a theme. *Anesthesiology* 1981; **55:** 335.

13. Gobbs C, Arandia H. A new technique for location and cannulation of the internal jugular vein. *Anesthesiology* 1981; **54:** 89.

14. Petty C. An alternate method for internal jugular venipuncture for monitoring venous pressure. *Anesthesia and Analgesia* 1975; **54:** 157.

15. Oshima E, Aria T, Urabe N. New anatomic landmarks for percutaneous catheterisation of the internal jugular vein. *Anesthesiology* 1991; **74:** 1164–6.

16. Chatrath RR, Stock JGL, Jones ODH. Internal jugular catheterisation in small children. *Anaesthesia* 1983; **38:** 381.

17. Nickalls RWD. A new percutaneous infraclavicular approach to the axillary vein. Infraclavicular approach to axillary vein. *Anaesthesia* 1987; **42:** 151–4.

18. Taylor BL, Yellowless I. Central venous cannulation using the infraclavicular axillary vein. *Anesthesiology* 1990; **72:** 55–8.

19. Smith MB, Till CWB. The axillary vein as an alternative. *Anaesthesia* 1994; **49:** 741–2.

20. Humphrey MJ, Blitt CD. Central venous access in children via the external jugular vein. *Anesthesiology* 1982; **57:** 50–1.

21. Scheller MS, Saidman LJ. An aid to identifying the external jugular vein. *Anesthesiology* 1982; **57:** 546–7.

22. Neustein SM, Narang J, Bronheim D. Use of the color test for safer internal jugular cannulation. *Anesthesiology* 1992; **76:** 1062.

23. Paw HGW. Tunnelling in the opposite direction. *Anaesthesia* 1996; **51:** 407–8.

24. Bailey CR. Tunnelling in the opposite direction. *Anaesthesia* 1996; **51:** 797–8.

25. Allen JG, Carter JA. Tunnelling technique for central venous catheters. *Anaesthesia* 1986; **41:** 770.

26. Gupta RM, Custer RM, Halim MY. An improved technique for antecubital central line placement. *Anesthesia and Analgesia* 1994; **79:** 604.

27. Gilston A. A teaching aid to venous and arterial pressure monitoring. *Anaesthesia* 1976; **31:** 554–6.

28. Fletcher SJ, Bodenham AR. Safe placement of central venous catheters: where should the tip of the catheter lie? *British Journal of Aanaesthesia* 2000; **85:** 188–91.

29. Fernandez-Cano F. A simple accurate technique for establishing zero reference levels for pressure measurements. *Anesthesiology* 1984; **61:** 478.

30. Knell PJW. Central venous pressure measurement *Anaesthesia* 1980; **35:** 991–2.

31. Worsley MH, Hawkins DJ, Scott DHT. Attachments to double lumen bronchial tube. *Anaesthesia* 1990; **45:** 1001–2.

Warming

Warming and maintaining body heat is important to

- increase patient comfort,

- maintain mental function,

- reduce oxygen demand, which in turn reduces the demand on the cardiac and respiratory systems,

- reduce sympathetic activity, shivering and hypoglycaemia.

Warming is achieved by adding heat using

- hot air overblanket,

- warm water or electric underblanket.

Conserve heat loss with

- metal foil sheet (light weight and convenient for resuscitation packs),

- large plastic (bin) bag which traps a layer of air between two layers of plastic.[1]

Warming intravenous fluids:

- An extension set should be fitted into a fluid warmer. An alternative is to gather up a length of extension tubing into three 8 in. loops and wrap them around the breathing tubing coming from the humidifier for infants or around a warming blanket for adults[2] (Figure 53).

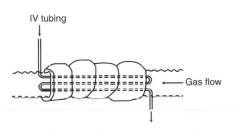

IV tubing

Gas flow

Figure 53 – Intravenous fluid warmer.

Weaning from Anaesthesia

Readiness for extubation postoperatively

There are usually four reasons why a patient may not breathe at the end of an operation:

- Low arterial carbon dioxide tension.

- Neuromuscular blockade.

- Sedation by opioids combined with other drugs.

- Breath holding due to the presence of the inflated cuff and tracheal tube in the trachea.

Steps to return to spontaneous breathing:

1. The arterial carbon dioxide will usually be above the normal 5.3 kPa before the patient breathes spontaneously due to the effect of anaesthetic drugs. This is achieved by rebreathing or adding carbon dioxide until an end-tidal CO_2 of 6–7 kPa is reached.

2. Assess neuromuscular function after non-depolarising drugs:

   - *Nerve stimulation.* Double burst stimulation of three stimuli at 50 Hz followed after 0.75 s by two or three stimuli at 50 Hz. There should be a contraction to the second stimulus before reversing the relaxant effect. A train of four stimuli at 2 Hz. The fourth stimulus should lead to a contraction before reversal is considered.

   - Inadequate reversal is suggested by jerky limb movements, difficulty in breathing and distress.

Treatment of partial paralysis:

- Sedate with midazolam 5–10 mg, to prevent the patient feeling partially paralysed.

W

- Hundred per cent oxygen and consider re-intubation if extubated.

- One to two litres of isotonic saline or Hartman's solution as rapidly as possible (5–10 min). This increases the volume of distribution of the drug and increases fluid flux at the neuromuscular junction.

- Do not administer a second dose of neostigmine. Doubling the dose of a drug does not double its effect. The first dose of neostigmine has already blocked the action of acetyl cholinesterase.

3. Effect of opioids. Give naloxone or a respiratory stimulant (doxopram) which may also reduce postoperative chest complications. Both drugs are short acting and the patient should be observed for the duration of the action of the opioid.

4. Breath holding on the tracheal tube and cuff. Perform laryngoscopy to inspect and clear pharynx of fluid then deflate the cuff.

If in doubt make sure the patient is responding to commands before extubation. Consider placing a tracheal suction catheter down the trachea before extubation to give oxygen and as a guide if re-intubation is necessary.

Predictors of successful weaning which have been suggested but are often difficult to put into practice in the recovering patient:

- Lifting the arm is a better test than lifting the head.

- Measurement of vital capacity and inspiratory force are recommended but difficult to achieve in the recovery patient. The patient's ability to inspire against a pressure of -18 cmH$_2$O at an air flow of 15 l/min is more theoretical than practical.[3]

- Tidal volume >5 ml/kg, FEV$_1$ >10 ml/kg, vital capacity >10–15 ml/kg, maximum inspiratory pressure >20–30 cmH$_2$O, minute ventilation <10 l/min and a maximum voluntary ventilation of twice the resting minute ventilation. It is also necessary to take into account the gag reflex and the ability or strength to cough.[4]

Weaning from long-term ventilation

Stop sedative drugs.

Opiates only for analgesia.

No paralysis or muscle weakness.

Assess ventilation to perfusion mismatch. Shunt <15% better <10%.

No organ in acute failure which is not controlled.

Deflate tracheal cuff.

Absence of tachypnoea or tachycardia.

Practical aids to weaning after longer periods of ventilation:

- Cuff deflation is an important step in improving upper airway function. Air passing through the larynx leads to better coordination of laryngeal and pharyngeal muscle function. It reduces the work of breathing by increasing the diameter of the airway.[5]

- Positive expiratory pressure. Expiration is normally associated with a closing of the larynx to generate a positive expiratory pressure. The worst time to assess oxygenation is on a T piece with no expiratory resistance.

- Inspiratory force of at least -40 cmH$_2$O, may be difficult to assess before extubation.

- Sustained eye opening.

- Hand grasp and tongue protrusion.

- Absence of tachycardia or tachypnoea, particularly in the elderly.

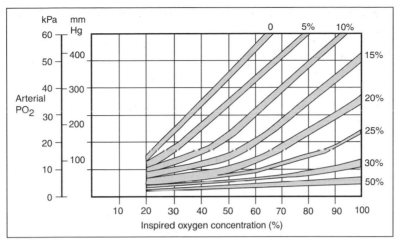

Figure 54 – Iso-shunt diagram.

• A ventilation to perfusion mismatch giving a shunt of less than 10% or less than a 5% increase on the preventilation shunt. Assessed using the iso-shunt diagram (Figure 54).

Nebulised local anaesthetic can be used to reduce tachypnoea and coughing and establish a normal pattern of breathing during weaning.[6]

Why do patients become hypoxic if weaned too early?

1. *Low alveolar oxygen.* Consider the alveolar air equation: $P_AO_2 = P_IO_2 - P_ACO_2/R$.

When breathing air the alveolar oxygen tension will be $20 - 5.3/0.8 = \sim14$ kPa. If the carbon dioxide tension rises to 8 as the patient hypoventilates, now $20 - 8/0.8 = 10$.

2. *Shunt:* The relationship between inspired oxygen tension and arterial oxygen tension can be plotted on an iso-shunt diagram.[7] The exact point on the diagram can be used to guide oxygen therapy. The trend in a series of readings gives an indicator of improvements in the patient's

condition. A virtual shunt of less than 10%, or within 5% of the shunt before the current illness is a good sign that weaning will be successful (Figure 54).

If the patient breathes 100% oxygen (100 kPa) but has an arterial oxygen tension of 15 kPa, and a carbon dioxide tension of 4 kPa then the alveolar oxygen tension will be $100 - 4/0.8 = 95$ kPa. The $A-a$ difference is $90 - 15 = 75$ (A difference of 2 kPa is normal breathing air or up to 15 kPa breathing 100% oxygen). The patient has a shunt of >25%. If the patient is now given 50% oxygen the alveolar oxygen would be $50 - 4/0.8 = 45$ kPa but the arterial tension will have dropped to 8 kPa or less, creating hypoxaemia. The hypoxaemia will be aggravated by any rise in carbon dioxide tension due to spontaneous respiration or exhaustion. If the P_ACO_2 rises to 8 kPa the equation becomes $P_AO_2 = 50 - 8/0.8 = 40$ kPa.

Weight and Obesity

A guide to an adult's weight in kg is their height in cm minus 100.

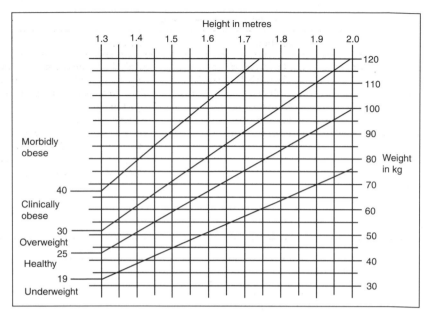

Figure 55 – Body mass index (from Garrow J.S. in obesity and related diseases 1988).

A child's weight is given by $(age + 4) \times 2$ in kg.

Body mass index = weight (kg)/height (m^2). In health this should be 19–25 for men, lower in women.

Obesity is a weight >20% above mean for age, or body mass index >30. Morbid obesity is a body mass index >40 (Figure 55).

To obtain a weight if it is off the scale

- Take two similar scales of equal weighing capacity placed side by side. The patient stands with one foot on each scale. The patient's weight is the sum of the weights taken at exactly the same time.

- Position one scale along side a platform at exactly the same height as the scale. The patient stands with one foot on the scale and one on the platform. The patient's weight (to be within 5%) is twice the weight on the scale.[8]

The problems of obesity include

- logistics;

- venous access;

- difficult airway and intubation;

- risk of DVT, bed sores, infection, accidental damage;

- increased oxygen demand increases cardiac output, hypertension, ischaemic heart disease, and stroke;

- increased respiratory effort but reduced FRC, breathlessness;

- regurgitate, hiatus hernia;

- diabetes mellitus;

- poor candidates for local blocks due to anatomy.

Weight and Obesity

Obesity checklist (with weight)

Anaesthesia	Medical	Logistics
Airway, short neck, difficult intubation	Hypertension	Difficulty in nursing due to limited mobility, turning and positioning
State of teeth	Myocardial ischaemia	Damage to skin: bed sore, nerves, pressure points
Snoring means airway obstruction	Diabetes	Venous thrombosis
Veins concealed and difficult to cannulate	Endocrine deficiencies	Monitoring — Difficulty
Titrate drugs for effect, not by weight	Regurgitation	BP — Correct cuff
Prevent hypoxia by preoxygenate, intubate, ventilate	Hiatus hernia	ECG — Electrode resistance
Postoperative oxygen		Pulse oximeter — Probe size

System	Effect
CVS	Increased oxygen demand Increased blood volume Increased cardiac work, cardiomegaly, atherosclerosis, coronary artery disease and hypertension; adipose tissue has low blood flow relative to mass
RS	Hypoxia due to Increased work of breathing Increased oxygen consumption and carbon dioxide production leading to hyperventilation Decreased vital capacity, functional residual capacity and compliance Increased shunt due to increased closing volume, within the tidal volume particularly when lying flat Diaphragmatic splinting
Renal	Renal function reduced Careful fluid balance due to reduced body water relative to weight
Endocrine	Glucose intolerance Diabetes Hypothyroidism
Surgery	Anatomy difficult Increased risk of wound infection Wound dehiscence
Risk of DVT, pulmonary embolism	Immobility Pressure on veins Dehydration
Bleeding	Increased
Anatomy	All procedures difficult: local and regional blocks, venous cannulation
Drugs	Abnormal response due to reduced body water relative to weight, high cardiac output

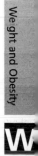

References

1. Ward ME. Cheap space blankets. *Anaesthesia* 1994; **49:** 182.
2. Rosen KR, Rosen DA, Broadman L. A simple method for warming intravenous fluid in infants. *Anesthesiology* 1986; **64:** 133.
3. Ibler M. Assessing inspiratory force – an indicator. *Anesthesiology* 1985; **62:** 695–6.
4. Shneerson JM. Are there new solutions to old problems with weaning. *British Journal of Anaesthesia* 1997; **78:** 238–40.
5. Bapat P, Verghese C. Cuff deflation for easier weaning from ventilation. *British Journal of Anaesthesia* 1997; **79:** 145.
6. Spivey K, Campbell D, Forrest F. Nebulised lignocaine: an aid to weaning. *Anaesthesia* 1994; **49:** 182.
7. Benatar SR, Hewlett AM, Nunn JF. The use of iso-shunt lines for control of oxygen therapy. *Anaesthesia* 1973; **45:** 711–18.
8. Foroughi V, Young M. What do you do when your patients outweigh your scales. *Anesthesia and Analgesia* 1995; **81:** 211–12.

Appendices

Drugs in Anaesthesia

Important anaesthetic drugs, effects, dose and use

Drug	Effect	Dose (IV)	Main use
Cardiovascular drugs			
Adrenaline (epinephrine)	Alpha high dose and beta low dose; increases heart rate, contractility, coronary blood flow, muscle dilatation	Bolus up to 1 mg, infusion 1–20 μg/min	Resuscitation, low cardiac output, asthma
Angiotensin (II)	Vasoconstrictor	1–20 μg/min	Hypotension
Dobutamine	Mostly beta$_1$, weak alpha	2–30 μg/kg/min	Low cardiac output
Dopamine	Alpha, beta, DA Low dose vasodilator High dose vasoconstrictor	Renal <2 μg/kg/min Cardiac 2–5 μg/kg/min Up to 20 μg/kg/min	Low cardiac output
Dopexamine	DA$_1$, DA$_2$, beta$_2$, less beta$_1$ vasodilator	0.5–3 μg/kg/min	Improve splanchnic blood flow
Ephedrine	Alpha and beta direct and indirect by releasing catecholamine; longer acting than epinephrine due to slower metabolism	5–15 mg/4 min	Hypotension
Noradrenaline (norepinephrine)	Alpha, less beta	15–250 ng/kg/min	Hypotension, increases coronary blood flow
Isoprenaline	Beta$_1$ and beta$_2$, increased heart rate and contractility	Solution 4 mg/ml, dose 0.01–0.1 μg/kg/min	Heart block
Metaraminol	Alpha and acetylcholine release	20–100 μg/kg/30 min	Hypotension
Methoxamine	Alpha, long acting, 1–2 h vasoconstrictor	Bolus 1–2 mg, infusion 1 μg/min	Hypotension
Atenolol	Beta-blocker, long acting, soluble does not cross to brain	1 mg/min up to 2.5 mg	Hypertension, angina, tachycardia
Amiodarone	Delays repolarisation by increasing duration of myocardial action potential; increases refractory period of atrial, nodal and ventricular tissue	5 mg/kg as 300 mg in 250 ml 5% glucose (not saline) 1200 mg/day	Arrhythmias, WPW syndrome
Digoxin	Increases contractility, slows conduction, arrhythmias, increases vagal effect	Bolus 10–15 μg/kg slowly, then 100 μg/day; check renal function and potassium	Atrial fibrillation, heart failure
Disopyramide	Reduces cardiac contractility anticholinergic, reduces effect of warfarin	5 mg/kg over 20–120 min maximum 1.2 g in 24 h	Ventricular arrhythmias
Esmolol	Beta-blocker, metabolised by plasma esterase so short acting	50–200 μg/kg/min	Early postmyocardial infarction

(Continued)

Drug	Effect	Dose (IV)	Main use
Labetalol	Beta-blocker and alpha$_1$, long 12 h action	2 mg/min up to 150 mg	Hypertension
Lidocaine	Negative inotrope and chronotrope, long acting	Boluses at 8 min intervals 0.5–250 mg/kg, infusion 2–4 mg/min	Ventricular arrhythmias

Antihypertensives
Propranolol	Beta-blocker	1 mg every few minutes	Tachycardia, angina, hypertension
Magnesium	Vasodilator, high dose monitor reflexes, respiration and serum level	4 g bolus IV, infusion 1 g/h or 4 g IV and 3 g IM to each buttock; target plasma level 4–6 mmol/l	Hypertension, eclampsia
Hydralazine	Vasodilator by arteriole muscle relaxation (not veins), reduces after load; this induces a sympathetic reflex, increases preload; avoid in angina	5–10 mg in 10 ml saline every 20 min; 200–300 µg/min reducing to 50 µg/min; limit 200 mg/day	Give with diuretic and beta-blocker in hypertension
Phenoxybenzamine	Irreversible alpha-blocker so long-acting vasodilator	Most require 1 mg/kg/day	Hypertension, phaeochromocytoma
Glyceryl trinitrate	Smooth muscle relaxant by NO; vasodilator, reduced preload	1–5 µg/kg/min	Vasoconstriction

Phosphodiesterase inhibitors
Enoximone	Increases active cyclic AMP, cardiac contractility	5–20 µg/kg/min	CCF
Milrinone	Increases active cyclic AMP	300–750 ng/kg/min	CCF

Anticonvulsants
Hemineverin (clomethiazole)		0.8% solution start 5 ml/min until fit stops, then 0.5–1 ml/min	Anticonvulsant
Phenytoin		10–15 mg/kg up to 50 mg/min, then 5–8 mg/kg/day	Anticonvulsant, ventricular arrhythmias
Diazemules	Facilitates GABA transmission, very long acting	Bolus 10 mg repeated, infusion 0.2–3 mg/kg/day	Anticonvulsant
Clonazepam	Benzodiazepine, less sedative, long active	1–3 mg	Anticonvulsant, muscle spasm

Respiratory stimulants
Doxopram	Stimulates; low dose carotid chemoreceptor, high dose medullary respiratory centre, action 10 min	Bolus 0.5–1.5 mg/kg, infusion 1–3 mg/min	

Diuretics
Frusemide	Loop diuretic, K$^+$ depletion	Infusion 2–4 mg/kg	Salt and water overload

153

(Continued)

Drug	Effect	Dose (IV)	Main use
Mannitol	Osmotic diuretic	10% or 20% solution 500 mg/kg	Water overload
DDAVP Desmopressin	Antidiuretic, little vasoconstriction, increases factor VIII	0.3 µg/kg	Diabetes insipidus, haemophilia and von Willebrand's disease
Prokinetic drugs			
Metoclopramide	Peripheral cholinergic agonist, increases gastric motility, relaxes pylorus, central dopamine antagonist	10 mg, large doses lead to dystonic muscle movements	Antiemetic, central effect and hastens gastric emptying
Domperidone	Does not easily cross blood brain barrier so little sedation or dystonia	10–20 mg po, 30 mg pr	Nausea and vomiting, abdominal distension
Antiemetics			
Haloperidol	Antagonist at domapine, serotonin, histamine and alpha receptors	Antiemetic 0.2–0.5 mg	Sedation, low dose antiemetic, schizophrenia
Phenothiazines	Sedation, antiemetic, antihistamine, vasodilator		
Cyclizine	Anticholinergic	50 mg	Opioid emesis
Ondansetron	Serotonin antagonist	4 mg repeated	Vomiting due to release of serotonin as in chemotherapy, bowel inflammation
Neuromuscular junction			
Suxamethonium	Depolarising relaxant	1–1.5 mg/kg	Effect prolonged by antibiotics, enzyme deficiencies
Mivacurium	Metabolised by pseudocholinesterase, short action	0.5–1 mg/kg	Non-depolarising muscle relaxant
Atracurium, bis-atracurium	30% Hoffman degradation limits action at 20 min	0.5 mg/kg	
Rocuronium		600 µg/kg, then 150 µg/kg/15 min or 500 µg/kg/h	
Vecuronium		80–100 µg/kg, then 20–30 µg/kg	
Pancuronium		50–100 µg/kg, then 10–20 µg/kg	
Neostigmine	Cholinesterase inhibitor, once enzyme is inhibited increased dose gives no further benefit; nicotinic and muscarinic effects	40–45 µg/kg with atropine 20 µg/kg	Reversal of non-depolarising relaxants
Physostigmine	As neostigmine but crosses blood brain barrier	14 µg/kg	Atropine and tricyclic poisoning

Drug	Effect	Dose (IV)	Main use
Atropine	Cholinergic antagonist	10–20 μg/kg 30+ μg/kg	Bradycardia Organophosphorus poisoning
Glycopyrronium	As atropine but less CNS and arrhythmia effect, potent antisialogogue	2–3 μg/kg	
Dantrolene	Peripherally acting muscle relaxant	2.4 mg/kg repeat after 15 min up to 10 mg/kg	Malignant hyperpyrexia
Respiratory system Salbutamol	Bronchodilator	Bolus 250 μg, infusion 3–20 μg/min	Bronchospasm, less tachycardia if inhaled
Aminophylline		Bolus 5 mg/kg over 20 min, infusion 500 μg/kg/h	Bronchospasm
Coagulation Heparin	Forms a complex with thrombin and antithrombin III which prevents fibrinogen forming fibrin	DVT prophylaxis 5000 units every 12 h, anticoagulation 300–600 units/kg/day	Measure KCCT, APTT
Haemofiltration Prostacyclin	For patients	2.5–5 ng/kg/min	During haemofiltration
Heparin fragmin	For circuits	200–600 units/h, 400 units/h	Coagulation screen daily
Sedation and analgesics Midazolam	Facilitates GABA transmissions	Bolus 10–300 μg/kg, infusion 1–3 μg/kg/min	Sedation, amnesia, anticonvulsant
Propofol	Anaesthesia (infusion – limit dose in children due to lipid load)	Bolus 2 mg/kg, infusion 10–200 mg/h	Sedation when rapid recovery required
Thiopentone	Reduces all CNS activity, apnoea, indirect vasodilator	Bolus 4 mg/kg, infusion 4–10 mg/kg/day	Anticonvulsant, sulphur link, reduces metabolic rate
Fentanyl	Analgesia and inhibits respiratory drive	Bolus 2–50 μg/kg, infusion 0.5–2 μg/kg/h	
Morphine	Analgesia	20–40 μg/kg/h	Mu, kappa and sigma agonist
Ketamine	Analgesia, sedation, hallucinations, sympathomimetic	1–2 mg/kg IV, always with anticholinergic and small dose benzodiazepine	Anaesthesia in difficult airway situations
Drugs of significance to anaesthetists Flumazenil	Inhibits benzodiazepine receptor, short action 1–3 h	Bolus usually up to 400 μg	Reversal of benzodiazepine effects
Naloxone	Antagonist at mu, kappa and sigma receptors	Start 100 μg	Reversal of opioid effects

155

(Continued)

Drug	Effect						Dose (IV)	Main use
Echothiophate	Long-acting anticholinesterase							Prolongs action of suxamethonium
Lithium	Long acting – days							Potentiates all muscle relaxants
Tricyclic antidepressants	Antagonist at acetylcholine, dopamine, serotonin and histamine receptors. Cardiac arrhythmias.							Use neurogenic pain in low doses. Anti-depressant higher doses
Volatile agents	MAC		SVP	Boiling	Solubility			
	50	90	(mmHg)	point (°C)	Blood/gas	Oil/gas		
Isoflurane	1.2	1.8	250	48.5	1.4	98		Vasodilator, hypotension
Enflurane	1.7	2.5	175	56	1.9	98		Similar but less CVS effects to halothane
Sevoflurane	2.0	3.0	160	58	0.7	53		Rapid induction and recovery
Halothane	0.7	1.5	243	50	2.3	224		Many CVS effects

Haematological and Biochemical Reference Values

Common haematology and biochemical values

	Adult male	Adult female	Child (2–12 years)
Haemoglobin	13.0–18.0	11.5–16.5	11.5–14.5 g/dl
Red cells	4.5–6.5	3.8–5.8	$4.0–5.4 \times 10^{12}/l$
Haematocrit	0.4–0.54	0.37–0.47	0.37–0.45
White cells	4.0–11.0		$4.5–13.5 \times 10^9/l$
Platelets	150–450		$150–450 \times 10^9/l$
MCV = PCV/red cells	80–96		75–96 fl
MCH = Hb/red cells	27–32		26–31 pg
MCHC = Hb/PCV	32–36		32–36 g/dl
Neutrophils	1.9–7.6		$1.5–8.5 \times 10^9/l$
Lymphocytes	1.3–4.0		$1.2–9.5 \times 10^9/l$
Monocytes	0.1–0.9		$0.1–0.9 \times 10^9/l$
Eosinophils	0–0.6		$0–0.7 \times 10^9/l$
Basophils	0–0.2		$0–0.1 \times 10^9/l$
Haematology			
Reticulocytes	$0.2–2.0\% (25–85 \times 10^9/l)$		
Plasma viscosity	1.50–1.72 mPa		
Vitamin B12	>170 ng/l		
Serum folate	>1.3 μg/l		
Red cell folate	>70 μg/l		
Ferritin	15–300 μg/l		
Haptoglobin	1–3 g/l		
Complement:			
C3	0.55–1.2 g/l		
C4	0.2–0.5 g/l		

(Continued)

	Adult male	Adult female
Antistreptolysin	A non-rising value of <200 IU/l	
Bleeding time	<10.5 min	
Prothrombin ratio (INR)	<1.2	
Partial thromboplastin time	40 s	
Thrombin time	+2 s on the control	
Fibrinogen	1.5–4.5 g/l	
INR therapeutic:		
Low-target range	2.0–3.0	
High-target range	3.0–4.0	
Heparin therapeutic range	90–120 s	
Fibrin degradation products	<10 mg/l	
D-dimer	<250 ng/l	
Protein S:		
Activity	70–150%	
Free	65–140%	
Total	70–160%	
Protein C:		
Activity	65–165%	
Antigen	75–155%	
Antithrombin III	80–155%	
Activated protein C resistance	>2.0 p	
Cardiolipin:		
IgG	<10 GPL U/ml	
IgM	<10 MPL U/ml	
Cold agglutinins:		
I cells	<1 in 64	
I cells	<1 in 16	
I enzyme cells	<1 in 128	
Haemoglobin A2	2.0–3.5%	
Haemoglobin F	<1%	
Biochemistry		
Sodium	130–155 mmol/l	
Potassium	3.0–5.5 mmol/l	
Urea	2.5 6.5 mmol/l	
Creatinine	80–120 mmol/l	
Glucose (random)	<8.0 mmol/l	
Chloride	98–108 mmol/l	
T CO_2	22–28 mmol/l	
T Protein	60–80 g/l	
Albumin	35–50 g/l	
Calcium	2.10–2.65 mmol/l	
Phosphate	0.8–1.4 mmol/l	
T bilirubin	5–17 mmol/l	
Cholesterol	<5.2 mmol/l	
CRP	<10 mg/l	
ALT	10–60 IU/l	
ALP	40–140 IU/l	
γ–GT	7–64 IU/l	
AST	10–42 IU/l	
CK	22–269 IU/l	
LDH	266–500 IU/l	

(Continued)

	Adult male	Adult female
Amylase		44–160 IU/l
FT3		3.5–6.5 pmol/l
FT4		10–23 pmol/l
TSH		0.35–5.50 μlU/ml
(H^+)		35–45 nmol/l
P_aO_2		12.0–13.3 kPa
P_aCO_2		4.9–5.9 kPa
Plasma Bicarb		24.0–32.0 mmol/l
BE		±2.0 mmol/l
$satO_2$		95–100%

Physiological Parameters

Cardiovascular values

Parameter	Normal value
Right atrial pressure	2–8 mmHg
Right ventricle pressure	0–40 mmHg
Pulmonary systolic artery pressure	16–24 mmHg
Pulmonary diastolic pressure	5–12 mmHg
Mean pulmonary artery pressure	9–16 mmHg
Pulmonary capillary wedge pressure	2–12 mmHg
Left atrial pressure	2–15 mmHg
Left ventricle pressure	0–140 mmHg
Systemic systolic/diastolic pressure	120/80 mmHg
Mean systemic pressure = (systolic pressure − diastolic pressure) × 1/3 + diastolic pressure	90–95 mmHg
Stroke volume	60–70 ml
Stroke index = stroke volume/surface area	40–50 ml/m^2
Ejection fraction = stroke volume/left ventricular volume	70%
Cardiac output = stroke volume × heart rate	70 × 70 ml/min or 70 ml/kg/min
Cardiac index = cardiac output/surface area, relates output to body size	2.5–3 l/min/m^2
Systemic vascular resistance = mean arterial pressure − right atrial pressure/cardiac output	$\frac{80 - 0}{5} = 10\text{–}15$ mmHg/l/min. Convert to cgs units (×80) 770–1500 dyne s/cm^5
Pulmonary vascular resistance = mean pulmonary artery pressure − wedge pressure/cardiac output	$\frac{16 - 8}{5} = 1.5\text{–}2.5$ mmHg/l/min cgs units = 120–200 dyne s/cm^5
Right cardiac work = right cardiac output × mean pulmonary artery pressure	5000 ml/min × 10 mmHg
Right cardiac work index = right cardiac work/surface area	0.54–0.66 kg min/m^2
Left cardiac work = left cardiac output × mean arterial pressure	5000 ml × 90 mmHg
Left cardiac work index = left cardiac work/surface area	3.4–4.2 kg min/m^2

Respiratory values

Parameter	Normal value
Minute ventilation = tidal volume × rate	5–7 l/min
Compliance = pressure required to achieve the tidal volume. Tidal volume/intrathoracic pressure − PEEP	25–35 ml/cmH$_2$O
Resistance = 1/compliance	0.3–1 cmH$_2$O/100 ml
Dead space = (P$_a$CO$_2$ − P$_E$CO$_2$) × tidal volume/P$_a$CO$_2$	145–155 ml 25–40% of tidal volume
Alveolar ventilation (tidal volume − dead space) × rate	4–5 l/min
Arterial oxygen content = Hb × 1.34 × arterial oxygen saturation/100 + (P$_a$O$_2$ × 0.0003 for O$_2$ in solution)	17–20 ml O$_2$/100 ml blood
Venous oxygen content = Hb × 1.34 × venous oxygen saturation/100 + (P$_v$O$_2$ × 0.0003)	12–15 ml/100 ml
Arterial venous difference	4.2–5 ml/100 ml
Oxygen availability = arterial oxygen content × cardiac output	900–1000 ml/min
Oxygen consumption = arterial venous difference × cardiac output	200–300 ml/min
Oxygen extraction ratio = ratio of oxygen consumed/oxygen available C$_a$O$_2$ − C$_v$O$_2$/C$_a$O$_2$	0.24–0.28
Carbon dioxide production	200–250 ml/min
Respiratory quotient = carbon dioxide produced/oxygen consumed (depends on diet)	0.7–1.0
Alveolar arterial difference. The effectiveness of oxygen exchange between alveoli and pulmonary capillary P$_A$O$_2$ − P$_a$O$_2$	5–15 mmHg breathing air
Breathing 100% oxygen. P$_A$O$_2$ = F$_i$O$_2$ × (barometric pressure − 47) − P$_a$CO$_2$	10–65 mmHg
Shunt Q$_s$/Q$_T$ = 100 × 1.34 × Hb + 0.0003 × P$_A$O$_2$ − C$_a$O$_2$/1.34 × Hb + 0.003 × P$_A$O$_2$ − C$_v$O$_2$	3–8%